The Flavorful Low-FODMAP Diet Cookbook

100 IBS-Friendly Recipes for Happy Digestion with Meal Plans, Food Intolerance Management, and FODMAP Elimination Strategies

Thomas O'Neal

Leave a review about our book:
As an independent author with a small marketing budget, reviews are my livelihood on this platform. If you enjoyed this book, I'd really appreciate it, if you left your honest feedback. You can do so by clicking review button.
I love hearing my readers and I personally read every single review!

Table of Contents

Chapter 1:

UNDERSTANDING THE LOW-FODMAP DIET

Embarking on the journey of understanding the Low-FODMAP Diet can be a transformative experience for those grappling with digestive issues such as irritable bowel syndrome (IBS). In this pivotal opening chapter, you will unravel the intricate science behind the Low-FODMAP Diet, demystifying the enigma of how certain fermentable carbohydrates can wreak havoc on your gut. Delve into the complexities of FODMAPs, from the oligosaccharides to the polyols, and unlock the knowledge of how these elusive culprits can trigger discomfort and abdominal bloating. Armed with this newfound comprehension, you will be empowered to seize control of your gut health and embark on a voyage towards enhanced digestive well-being. Bid farewell to the bewilderment and exasperation of managing your digestive symptoms, and brace yourself to learn about Low-FODMAP Diet by reading through the text of this chapter!

What Are FODMAPs?

"Fermentable Oligosaccharides, Disaccharides, Monosaccharides, and Polyols, or FODMAPS," are collectively recognized as small or short-chained carbohydrates that are naturally present in some food items. FODMAPs are known to be poorly absorbed in a person's small intestine and can cause symptoms in some individuals with sensitive digestive systems. FODMAPs are present in a variety of foods. Some examples of specific types of FODMAPs include:

- **Oligosaccharides**: Fructans and galacto-oligosaccharides (GOS), which are present in foods such as rye, wheat, garlic, onions, and legumes (e.g., lentils and chickpeas).
- **Disaccharides**: Lactose, which is present in milk and dairy food items.
- **Monosaccharides**: One good example is fructose, which is present in some varieties of honey, fructose-rich corn syrup and fruits.
- **Polyols**: Sorbitol, mannitol, xylitol, and maltitol, which are sugar alcohols found in some fruits, vegetables, and artificial sweeteners.

How Does Low-FODMAP Diet Works?

The utilization of this diet is considered as a viable strategy for addressing symptoms linked to irritable bowel syndrome (IBS) and other gastrointestinal ailments. This approach entails a temporary restriction or reduction of foods high in FODMAPs, which are types of small or short-chain carbs and sugar alcohols that have been implicated in triggering digestive symptoms in certain individuals. The low-FODMAP diet is typically conducted in three distinct phases, including the elimination period, the reintroduction phase, and the maintenance phase, each serving a unique purpose in the management of symptoms.

Elimination Phase: It lasts for 2 to 6 weeks, in which all the high-FODMAP items are Taken off the diet. This phase aims to reduce the overall FODMAP load in the diet and alleviate digestive symptoms. Common high-FODMAP foods that are eliminated during this phase include onions, garlic, wheat, rye, certain fruits and vegetables, dairy products, and some artificial sweeteners. The diet is typically followed strictly during this phase.

Reintroduction Phase: After the elimination phase, individual FODMAPs are systematically introduced back into the diet, one by one, to pin down which specific FODMAPs trigger symptoms in an individual. This phase helps to determine a person's tolerance to different FODMAPs and identify their specific trigger foods. The reintroduction phase is done under the guidance of a qualified healthcare professional, and symptoms are carefully monitored and recorded during this phase.

Maintenance Phase: The maintenance phase involves personalizing the diet by including a variety of low-FODMAP and tolerated foods while avoiding or minimizing the intake of high-FODMAP foods that trigger symptoms. This phase aims to create a sustainable long-term dietary plan that meets the individual's nutritional needs while managing their digestive symptoms.

Getting Started On Low-FODMAP Diet

Starting a low-FODMAP dietary approach must ideally be done under the advice and guidance of a qualified healthcare professional, such as a registered dietitian or gastroenterologist, who can provide personalized recommendations based on your individual needs and health condition. However, here are some general steps to get started on a low-FODMAP diet:

Educate Yourself: Familiarize yourself with the list of high-FODMAP items to avoid and low-FODMAP items that are safe to consume. There are many online resources, books, and apps that provide detailed information on the Low-FODMAP Diet.

Plan Your Meals: Create a meal plan that includes low-FODMAP foods for each meal and snack. This can help you stay organized and ensure you have suitable options available. There are several meal planning apps and websites that can assist you in creating Low-FODMAP meal plans.

Read Food Labels: Be diligent about reading food labels to identify high-FODMAP ingredients. Avoid foods that contain ingredients rich in galactans, lactose, fructans, fructose, and polyols. Look for Low-FODMAP certified labels on food products, as some companies now provide specific Low-FODMAP labeling.

Shop Smart: Make a grocery list before you go shopping and stick to it. Focus on buying fresh fruits, vegetables, meats, and grains that are low in FODMAP. Avoid processed and pre-packaged foods, as they often contain high-FODMAP ingredients. Shop in the periphery of the grocery store, where you will found fresh produce, meats, and dairy.

Plan for Snacks: Stock up on low-FODMAP snacks such as rice cakes, nuts, seeds, hard cheeses, carrots, cucumbers, and low-FODMAP fruits like berries or oranges. Having these snacks readily available can help you resist the temptation of high-FODMAP options.

Experiment with Recipes: There are plenty of delicious Low-FODMAP recipes available online. Experiment with different recipes and find ones that suit your tastes and dietary preferences. Cooking at home allows you to have full control over the ingredients and portion sizes.

Keep a Food Diary: Keeping a food diary can help you track your symptoms and identify any potential trigger foods. Jot down what you eat, when you eat it, and any symptoms you experience. This can help you identify patterns and make adjustments to your diet as desired.

Be Mindful of Portion Sizes: While a food may be low-FODMAP in small quantities, consuming large amounts may still trigger symptoms. Pay close attention to portion sizes and avoid overeating, especially with high-FODMAP foods.

Be Patient: It may take time to see improvements in your symptoms after starting the low-FODMAP Diet. Everyone's body is different, and it may take some errors to find the right approach that works for you. Be patient, keep track of your progress, and work closely with your registered dietitian to make necessary adjustments.

Macronutrients

Macronutrients refer to the three main types of nutrients that our body needs in large amounts for energy and overall functioning: carbohydrates, proteins, and fats. While trying a low-FODMAP diet, it's crucial to ensure that you're still getting a balanced intake of macronutrients to meet your body's energy needs. This may involve choosing low-FODMAP sources of carbohydrates, such as rice or quinoa, lean proteins like chicken or fish, and healthy fats like avocado or nuts.

Micronutrients

Micronutrients are essential nutrients that our body needs in smaller amounts but are crucial for maintaining overall health. These include vitamins and minerals such as vitamin D, vitamin C, magnesium, and zinc. While on a FODMAP diet, it's important to pay attention to getting a variety of low-FODMAP foods that are rich in micronutrients to support optimal health and prevent nutrient deficiencies.

Fiber

It is an important nutrient that plays a major role in gut health and digestive function. However, some high-fiber foods can be high in FODMAPs and may trigger symptoms in individuals with certain digestive issues. It's important to choose low-FODMAP sources of fiber, such as carrots, cucumbers, or gluten-free oats, to maintain adequate fiber intake while on a FODMAP diet.

Calcium

Calcium is an essential mineral that is important for your bone health, nerve function, and muscle contraction. Some common sources of calcium, such as dairy products, may be limited on a FODMAP diet due to lactose intolerance. However, there are still low-FODMAP options for calcium, such as lactose-free dairy items, fortified plant-sourced milk, or low-lactose cheeses like cheddar or Swiss.

Iron

It is a mineral that is necessary for producing red blood cells in the body and carrying oxygen throughout the body. While some high-iron foods, such as legumes or lentils, may be limited on a FODMAP diet, there are still low-FODMAP sources of iron available, including lean meats, fish, poultry, and fortified gluten-free cereals.

Hydration

Water intake is important for maintaining regular bowel movements and preventing constipation, which can be a common issue for those following a FODMAP diet. It's important to prioritize hydration and drink plenty of water throughout the day, especially if you are increasing your fiber intake or experiencing digestive symptoms.

Chapter 2:

LIVING A LOW-FODMAP LIFESTYLE

Living a low-FODMAP lifestyle can be a game-changer for those suffering from digestive issues. By following a low-FODMAP diet, you have the power to take control of your gut health, reduce uncomfortable symptoms such as bloating, gas, and pain in the abdomen, and improve your overall quality of life. Imagine being able to enjoy your meals without the fear of triggering your digestive system and feeling more energized and confident in your daily activities. With a low-FODMAP lifestyle, you have the opportunity to unlock the true potential of your body and experience a new level of wellness, allowing you to thrive and fully embrace life to the fullest. Say goodbye to digestive discomfort and hello to a world of culinary possibilities where you can savor delicious foods without compromise. Embrace the empowering journey of living a low-FODMAP lifestyle, and open the door to a healthier, happier you.

Managing Stress And Anxiety

Managing stress and anxiety is crucial for overall well-being, and it becomes even more important when you are following a low-FODMAP lifestyle to counter irritable bowel syndrome (IBS) or similar gastrointestinal problems.

The Relationship Between Stress, Anxiety, and IBS
The relationship between stress, anxiety, and irritable bowel syndrome (IBS) is complicated and multifactorial. While stress and anxiety do not directly cause IBS, they can worsen IBS symptoms and trigger flare-ups in individuals who are susceptible to gastrointestinal issues.

Stress and anxiety can impact the functioning of the gastrointestinal tract through the brain-gut connection, which is a bidirectional communication network between the brain and the gut. Our gut has its own "nervous system," which is named as enteric nervous system (ENS), referred to as the "second brain," which communicates with the brain's central nervous system (CNS). Stress and anxiety can disrupt the normal functioning of the brain-gut connection, which leads to alterations in gut motility, increased sensitivity to pain, and changes in gut immune function, which can trigger or exacerbate IBS symptoms.

Additionally, stress and anxiety can also affect behaviors and coping mechanisms that may impact IBS symptoms. For example, stress and anxiety can lead to changes in eating patterns, such as skipping meals, emotional eating, or consuming trigger foods, which can worsen IBS symptoms in susceptible individuals. Stress and anxiety can also lead to changes in sleep patterns, reduced physical activity, and altered social interactions, which can all contribute to IBS symptom exacerbation.

Simple Techniques for Managing Stress

Managing stress and anxiety is, therefore, an important aspect of managing IBS symptoms. By practicing stress controlling techniques, like mindfulness, exercise, and seeking support from friends, family, or professionals, individuals with IBS can potentially reduce the impact of stress and anxiety on their gut health and overall well-being.

Prioritize self-care: Make self-care a priority in your daily routine. This can include activities such as exercise, getting quality sleep, practicing techniques to relax like meditation or deep breathing, engaging in hobbies, spending time with loved ones, and doing things that bring you joy and relaxation.

Identify and manage triggers: Be aware of situations or factors that trigger stress or anxiety for you. It could be work-related stress, family issues, financial concerns, or other personal challenges.

Plan and prepare meals in advance: Meal planning and preparation can help you stay organized and reduce stress around meal times. Plan and prepare your low-FODMAP meals and snacks in advance so you have suitable options readily available. This can help you avoid last-minute stress and anxiety about finding suitable foods to eat.

Practice mindfulness: Mindfulness is a powerful technique to manage stress and anxiety. Practice being present at the moment and fully engaging in activities without judgment. This can aid you in becoming more aware of your mental thoughts and emotions and better at managing stress and anxiety when they arise.

Stay connected: Social support is crucial for managing stress and anxiety. Stay connected with friends, family, or support groups who understand your challenges with a low-FODMAP lifestyle. Share your thoughts and feelings with them and seek their support when needed.

Get regular exercise: Physical activity serves as a natural antidote to stress, working wonders to uplift your mood and alleviate anxiety. By integrating a consistent exercise regimen into your daily routine, whether it's walking, jogging, practicing yoga, or engaging in any other form of enjoyable physical activity that aligns with your health condition, you can experience the remarkable benefits it brings.

Get enough sleep: Sleep is essential for managing stress and anxiety. Make sure you prioritize getting enough restful sleep each night. Create a calming bedtime routine, avoid stimulating activities before sleep time, and create a comfortable sleep environment to support quality sleep.

Mindfulness and Relaxation Exercises

Practicing mindfulness and relaxation exercises can be beneficial in managing stress and anxiety, which in turn can help avoid triggering or worsening irritable bowel syndrome (IBS) symptoms. Here are some techniques you can try:

Deep breathing: Find a quiet place, sit comfortably, and take deep and slow breaths in through your nose, allowing your belly to expand. Then exhale slowly through your mouth, letting go of any tension or stress with each breath.

Progressive muscle relaxation: Progressive muscle relaxation includes tensing and relaxing different groups of muscles in the body to release tension and promote relaxation. Start by tensing one muscle group, such as your shoulders or hands, and then release the tension while taking slow, deep breaths. Move through different muscle groups in your body, focusing on one at a time to help relax your entire body.

Mindful meditation: Mindful meditation involves focusing on the present moment without judgment. Find a quiet place, sit comfortably, and focus your attention on your breath or a specific sensation in your body. Notice any thoughts or emotions that arise, without judgment, and gently bring your focus back to the present moment.

Guided imagery: Guided imagery involves using your imagination to create calming mental images. You can use pre-recorded guided imagery sessions or create your own by visualizing a peaceful scene, like sitting on a beach or walking through a forest, and imagining yourself being present in that scene. Engaging your senses in the imagery can help you relax and reduce stress.

Body scan: It involves systematically introducing awareness to different parts of your body and noticing any feeling or sensation, without judgment. Lie down in a comfortable position, then close your eyes, and start with your toes, moving slowly up through your body, paying attention to each body part and any sensations you may feel.

Yoga or Tai Chi: Yoga and Tai Chi are physical activities that incorporate relaxation techniques, mindfulness, and gentle movements. These practices can help enhance flexibility, strength, and balance while also aiding relaxation and stress reduction.

The Role of Exercise in Stress Reduction

Exercise plays a vital role in reducing stress, with regular physical activity being shown to be a natural and effective stress reliever that can greatly improve mental well-being. One of the ways exercise can alleviate stress is through the release of endorphins. When we exercise, our brain releases chemicals called endorphins, which are our natural painkillers and mood elevators. These endorphins can help improve our mood, reduce anxiety, and supports an overall sense of well-being, thus helping to alleviate stress.

Exercise also helps in reducing stress hormones in the body. Stress hormones like cortisol and adrenaline are known to contribute to chronic stress. Regular exercise can help regulate the levels of these hormones, reducing their impact on the body and helping to manage stress more effectively. Another way in which exercise can help reduce stress is by improving sleep quality. Regular exercise has been shown to enhance sleep quality, which is essential for overall well-being and stress reduction. Better sleep can help reduce irritability, fatigue, and mood swings, all of which are common symptoms of stress.

Staying Motivated and Consistent

Maintaining motivation and consistency in a FODMAP lifestyle can be truly transformative for individuals grappling with digestive problems. Envision a life where you can savor your favorite foods without enduring distressing symptoms. Envision yourself feeling invigorated, harmonious, and unencumbered by digestive discomfort. By steadfastly adhering to a FODMAP lifestyle, you are taking charge of your health and well-being. Each day that you choose to adhere to the FODMAP guidelines, you are making a positive investment in your own physical health, bestowing upon yourself the invaluable gift of improved gut health.

Tracking Your Symptoms and Progress
Tracking your symptoms and the progress of a Low-FODMAP lifestyle can be a helpful tool in managing irritable bowel syndrome (IBS) and identifying triggers for your symptoms. Here are some tips for tracking your symptoms and progress:

Keep a symptom journal

Start by keeping a journal to record your IBS symptoms, like pain in the abdomen, gas, diarrhea, constipation, or bloating. Note the severity and duration of each symptom, as well as any potential triggers, such as specific foods, stress levels, or other factors that may affect your symptoms. You can use a paper journal or a digital tool such as a note-taking app or a symptom-tracking app to record your symptoms on a daily basis.

Record your diet

Since you are following a Low-FODMAP lifestyle, it's important to track your diet to identify any potential trigger foods or patterns. Keep a record of the foods you eat, including portion sizes, and note any symptoms that occur after each meal or snack. This can help you identify which foods may be causing your symptoms and make adjustments to your diet accordingly.

Monitor stress levels

Stress can be a major trigger for IBS symptoms, so it's important to monitor your stress levels as well. Record your stress levels in your symptom journal, noting any stressful events or situations that may have occurred during the day. This can help you identify patterns between stress and your symptoms and take steps to manage stress more effectively.

Track lifestyle factors

In addition to diet and stress, other lifestyle factors can also impact your IBS symptoms. Keep track of factors such as sleep patterns, physical activity levels, medication use, and any other relevant lifestyle factors. This can help you identify any patterns or correlations between these factors and your symptoms.

Assess progress

Regularly review your symptom journal to assess your progress over time. Look for any trends or patterns in your symptoms, diet, stress levels, and lifestyle factors. Identify any of your triggers or patterns that may be contributing to your symptoms, and use this information to make adjustments to your low-FODMAP lifestyle, such as avoiding trigger foods, managing stress, or making other lifestyle changes.

Developing Healthy Habits for Long-Term Success

Developing healthy habits for long-term success on a low-FODMAP lifestyle is the key to unlocking sustained relief from digestive issues. It's about more than just following a short-term diet - it's about cultivating a lasting lifestyle that nurtures your gut health and overall well-being. By consistently integrating FODMAP-friendly foods into your daily routine, prioritizing mindful eating, staying hydrated, and maintaining regular physical activity, you are laying the foundation for a healthier future. These small yet powerful habits can help you maintain balance, reduce symptoms, and enjoy a higher quality of life in the long run. It's not just about temporary fixes but about creating sustainable routines that become second nature. With patience, determination, and a commitment to self-care, you can develop healthy habits that will support your low-FODMAP lifestyle for the long haul, empowering you to thrive and enjoy a lifetime of digestive wellness. Your gut health deserves nothing less than your unwavering dedication to long-term success!

- **Create a meal plan:** Planning your meals in advance can help you make informed food choices and make sure that you are consistently following a low-FODMAP diet. Create a meal plan for the week that includes low-FODMAP foods, and make a grocery list accordingly. Having a full-fledged plan in place can help you stay on track and avoid impulsive food choices that may trigger your symptoms.
- **Cook at home:** Cooking your meals at home gives you better control over the ingredients and portion sizes, allowing you to maintain a low-FODMAP diet more effectively. Experiment with low-FODMAP recipes and meal prep to make healthy and delicious meals at home.
- **Stay organized**: Keeping your kitchen organized and stocked with Low-FODMAP foods can make it easier to stick to your low-FODMAP lifestyle. Label your pantry items, fridge, and freezer to easily identify low-FODMAP foods. Keep a list of low-FODMAP foods and snacks handy for

quick reference, and declutter your kitchen to create a clean and organized space for food preparation.

- **Practice portion control:** Paying attention to portion sizes can aid you in maintaining a healthy diet and preventing overeating, which can trigger IBS symptoms. Use quality measuring cups or a food scale to ensure that you are consuming appropriate portions of low-FODMAP foods. Avoid eating large meals or heavy snacks close to bedtime, as this can contribute to discomfort and disrupt sleep.

- **Stay hydrated**: Drinking lots of water and healthy fluids throughout the day is essential for overall health and can also help with digestion. Aim to drink plenty of water and stay hydrated, as dehydration can worsen constipation or diarrhea, which are common symptoms of IBS. Carry a water bottle with you to remind yourself to drink water regularly.

- **Practice stress management techniques**: Stress can exacerbate IBS symptoms, so it's important to develop a healthy stress management mechanism. Add relaxation techniques to your routine, such as deep breathing exercises, meditation, or yoga, into your daily routine. Regular exercise and getting enough sleep are also important for managing stress and supporting overall well-being.

Chapter 3:

FODMAP-FRIENDLY INGREDIENTS

This chapter on FODMAP-Friendly Ingredients is a treasure trove for those following a low-FODMAP diet. Packed with delicious and nutritious options, this chapter is a culinary guide that empowers you to create flavorful and satisfying meals without triggering your digestive symptoms. From gluten-free grains and low-FODMAP fruits and vegetables to protein-rich meats, poultry, and seafood, this chapter is a comprehensive resource for selecting ingredients that are gentle on your gut. You'll discover creative ways to use lactose-free dairy, dairy alternatives, firm tofu, nuts, and seeds to add protein and texture to your dishes. With practical tips on ingredient swaps, portion sizes, and cooking techniques, this chapter will help you navigate the world of FODMAP-friendly ingredients with confidence, opening up a world of culinary possibilities while keeping your digestive comfort in mind.

Understanding FODMAPs and Ingredient Selection

FODMAPs have the potential to attract water into the intestines and undergo rapid fermentation by gut bacteria. This can lead to the manifestation of various uncomfortable symptoms such as excessive gas, bloating, pain in the abdomen, diarrhea, and/or constipation. To alleviate these gastrointestinal issues, a short-term elimination diet known as the low-FODMAP diet is often suggested, which involves avoiding foods that are high in FODMAPs to reduce the intake of these fermentable carbohydrates. Choosing the right Ingredients when following a low-FODMAP diet is crucial to ensure that the meals are well-tolerated and do not trigger symptoms. Here are some tips for selecting FODMAP-friendly ingredients:

Look for alternative sources of flavor: Since many high-FODMAP ingredients, such as onions, garlic, and certain spices, are commonly used for flavoring in cooking, it's important to look for alternative sources of flavor. For example, you can use herbs such as basil, oregano, thyme, or rosemary to add flavor to your meals without adding FODMAPs.

Avoid processed foods: Processed foods can contain hidden sources of FODMAPs, such as high-fructose corn syrup, fructooligosaccharides (FOS), or inulin, which are commonly used as sweeteners or bulking agents. It's important to carefully read ingredient labels and pick minimally processed, whole foods as much as possible to reduce the risk of consuming hidden FODMAPs.

Pay attention to serving sizes: Some foods may be low in FODMAPs when consumed in small amounts, but can become high in FODMAPs when consumed in larger quantities. It's imperative to pay attention to serving sizes and portion control, especially for foods that are moderate in FODMAPs, to avoid overconsumption of FODMAPs.

Be mindful of fruit and vegetable choices: Fruits and vegetables can be major contributors to FODMAPs in the diet. It's important to choose low-FODMAP options and be mindful of portion sizes. For example, bananas, blueberries, strawberries, grapes, oranges, and pineapple are generally well-tolerated low-FODMAP fruits, while high-FODMAP fruits such as apples, cherries, watermelon, and mangoes should be avoided or consumed in a trace amount.

Experiment with alternative Ingredients: There are many alternative ingredients that can be used in a low-FODMAP diet to replace high-FODMAP foods. For example, you can use garlic-infused oil instead of garlic, scallion greens instead of onion, and lactose-free dairy products instead of regular dairy products.

Keep a food diary: Keeping a food diary and recording your symptoms can help you identify which foods trigger your symptoms and which Ingredients are well-tolerated. This can be helpful in fine-tuning your low-FODMAP diet and identifying any potential sources of hidden FODMAPs.

FODMAP-Friendly Protein
This nutrient is indispensable for the body as it has a pivotal role in tissue building, tissue repair, immune system support, and energy provision. Even if you are adhering to a low-FODMAP diet, you can still indulge in a diverse range of protein sources that are considered compatible with the diet's guidelines. Here are some examples:

- **Meat and poultry**: The majority of meat and poultry options are inherently low in FODMAPs and can be safely incorporated into a diet that follows low-FODMAP guidelines. Examples include beef, pork, lamb, chicken, and turkey. It's important to choose unprocessed or minimally processed cuts of meat, as some processed meats may contain high-FODMAP Ingredients such as garlic or onion powder.
- **Seafood:** Seafood is generally low in FODMAPs and can be a great source of protein in a low-FODMAP diet. Examples include fish, shrimp, crab, lobster, and scallops. However, it's important to avoid high-FODMAP seafood such as clams, mussels, and oysters.
- **Eggs**: Eggs are a versatile and nutrient-rich source of protein and are considered low in FODMAPs. They can be incorporated into various dishes, including omelets, frittatas, and egg-based casseroles.

- **Firm tofu**: Firm tofu is a low-FODMAP plant-based protein source that can be used in a variety of dishes. It's important to choose firm tofu, as soft or silken tofu may contain higher levels of FODMAPs.
- **Lactose-free dairy or dairy alternatives**: Dairy products that are lactose-free, such as milk, yogurt, and cheese, along with non-dairy alternatives like almond, coconut, and rice milk (labeled as low-FODMAP), can serve as suitable sources of protein in a diet that adheres to low-FODMAP principles.
- **Nuts and seeds**: Both nuts and seeds are recognized for their low-FODMAP content, making them viable protein options in a diet that follows low-FODMAP guidelines. Examples of suitable choices include almonds (whole or cut up), walnuts, chia, sunflower, and pumpkin seeds. However, it is essential to avoid nuts and seeds that are high in FODMAPs, such as cashews, pistachios, and sesame seeds.

FODMAP-Friendly Carbohydrates

FODMAPs carbohydrates are improperly absorbed in the small intestine, which leads to potential digestive discomfort for some individuals. However, not all carbohydrates are high in FODMAPs. There are several FODMAP-friendly carbohydrates that can be included in a low-FODMAP diet. Here are some examples:

1. **Gluten-free grains**: Quinoa, rice (including white, brown, basmati, and jasmine), cornmeal, polenta, oats (if labeled as gluten-free), and gluten-free pasta (made from rice, corn, or quinoa) are generally low in FODMAPs and can be included to your low-FODMAP diet.

2. **Low-FODMAP fruits**: Some fruits are considered low in FODMAPs and can be enjoyed in moderation. Examples include strawberries, blueberries, raspberries, grapes, oranges, kiwi, and pineapple. It's crucial to take care of the portion sizes and choose ripe fruits, as unripe fruits can be higher in FODMAPs.

3. **Low-FODMAP vegetables:** Many vegetables can be included in a low-FODMAP diet, including carrots, bell peppers, cucumbers, lettuce, spinach, zucchini, eggplant, green beans, and tomatoes (excluding cherry tomatoes). Avoid high-FODMAP vegetables like onions, garlic, and mushrooms.

4. **Low-FODMAP sweeteners**: Some sweeteners are considered low in FODMAPs and can be used in small quantities. Examples include maple syrup, rice malt syrup, stevia, and glucose syrup. However, it's crucial to avoid sweeteners like agave syrup, honey, and fructose-rich corn syrup, which are high in FODMAPs.

FODMAP-Friendly Fats

Olive oil: It is a healthy fat that is well-tolerated on a low-FODMAP diet. Use it for cooking, drizzling over salads, or as a base for homemade dressings and sauces.

Avocado: Avocado is a delicious and nutritious source of healthy fats that is generally low in FODMAPs. It can be mashed and used as a spread, put into salads, or used as a topping for various dishes.

Nuts and seeds: Several nuts and seeds are low in FODMAPs and can be taken in moderation on your low-FODMAP diet. Options include almonds, walnuts, pecans, chia seeds, and flaxseeds. They can be used as a topping for salads, put into smoothies, or eaten as a snack.

Coconut oil: Coconut oil is a source of healthy fats that can be used in cooking and baking. It is low in FODMAPs and can be used as an alternative to other cooking oils in low-FODMAP recipes.

Chapter 4:

FOOD INTOLERANCE MANAGEMENT SCIENCES

Managing food intolerances, such as FODMAP sensitivity, requires careful planning and strategic approaches. The key to success lies in learning and understanding your body's unique response to certain foods and implementing effective management strategies. This may involve keeping a food diary to track trigger foods, following an elimination diet approach to identify intolerances, and gradually reintroducing high-FODMAP foods during the reintroduction phase. It also includes adopting coping strategies for common digestive issues, such as bloating and gas, constipation, and diarrhea, through dietary adjustments, lifestyle modifications, and proper hydration and fiber intake.

Identifying Trigger Foods

Keeping a detailed food diary can help identify patterns and pinpoint specific foods that may be causing discomfort. By carefully observing your body's response to different foods, you can determine which high-FODMAP foods are triggering your symptoms and make informed decisions about what to include or avoid in your diet. Identifying trigger foods is an essential first step in developing a personalized and effective FODMAP management plan.

Understanding Food Intolerance vs. Allergy
Food intolerance refers to the body's inability to digest or absorb certain foods properly, leading to symptoms like bloating, gastric issues, diarrhea, and pain in abdomen. On the other hand, food allergy is an immune response triggered by specific proteins in foods, leading to symptoms such as hives, swelling, difficulty breathing, and in severe cases, anaphylaxis.

Keeping a Food Diary
Keeping a food diary is a crucial step in identifying trigger foods on a FODMAP diet. It involves documenting all the foods and beverages consumed, along with any associated symptoms, in a journal or an app. This helps in tracking the connection between the intake of certain food items and the onset of certain symptoms and can provide valuable insights into identifying potential trigger foods. The food diary should be maintained consistently for a period of time, typically 2-4 weeks, to gather enough data for analysis.

Elimination Diet Approach
The elimination diet approach is a key strategy used in the FODMAP diet to identify trigger foods. It involves eliminating all high-FODMAP foods from your diet for a certain period of time, usually 2-6 weeks. High-FODMAP foods are those that are known to contain high levels of fermentable carbohydrates that may trigger symptoms in sensitive individuals.

Importance of Reintroduction Stage
After the elimination stage, the reintroduction stage is a crucial step in identifying specific trigger foods for an individual. In this phase, high-FODMAP food items are systematically introduced back into the diet one by one, in controlled amounts, while monitoring symptoms using the food diary. This helps to identify which specific FODMAPs or foods are triggering symptoms in the individual, as different people may have different trigger foods.

Common Trigger Foods and their FODMAP Levels
There are several common trigger foods that are known to be high in FODMAPs and may cause symptoms in individuals with FODMAP intolerance. Some examples of high-FODMAP foods and their corresponding FODMAP levels include:

- Fructans: present in wheat, onions, garlic, and some fruits, such as apples and pears.
- Lactose: present in dairy products like yogurt, milk, and soft cheeses.
- Fructose: present in honey, high-fructose corn syrup, and certain fruits, such as apples, pears, and watermelon.
- Polyols: found in sugar alcohols, such as sorbitol, mannitol, xylitol, and certain fruits, such as avocados, cherries, and stone fruits.

Coping with Digestive Issues

Are you tired of struggling with uncomfortable bloating, gas, constipation, or diarrhea? Coping with digestive issues can be challenging, but there are effective strategies to help you take control of your gut health. From managing your diet and staying hydrated to incorporating gut-healing foods and natural remedies, you can find relief and improve your overall well-being. Don't let digestive issues hold you back from enjoying life to the fullest. Discover the strategies that work best for you and take steps towards a healthier gut today!

Strategies for Managing Bloating and Gas
Bloating and gas are common digestive symptoms that can be experienced by individuals following a FODMAP diet. Here are some strategies for managing bloating and gas:

a. Avoiding high-FODMAP foods: As per the FODMAP diet, avoiding or limiting the intake of high-FODMAP foods such as onions, garlic, legumes, and certain fruits can help reduce bloating and gas in sensitive individuals.

b. Eating smaller, more frequent meals: Eating smaller and frequent meals, instead of 2-3 large meals, can help reduce the risk of bloating and gas. Overeating can put extra pressure on the digestive system, leading to increased gas production.

c. Chewing food thoroughly: Properly chewing food helps break it down before swallowing, which can aid in digestion and reduce the amount of gas produced in the gut.

d. Avoiding carbonated beverages and chewing gum: Carbonated beverages and chewing gum can introduce excess air into the digestive system, leading to increased gas production and bloating. Limiting or avoiding these can help manage bloating and gas.

Dealing with Constipation and Diarrhea

Constipation and diarrhea are other common digestive issues that individuals may experience while following a FODMAP diet. Here are some strategies for managing constipation and diarrhea:

- Ensuring adequate water intake: Staying hydrated is important for maintaining regular bowel movements. Drinking lots of water during the day can help soften stools and ease constipation, as well as prevent dehydration in case of diarrhea.
- Incorporating low-FODMAP fiber sources: Adequate fiber intake is important for maintaining regular bowel movements. Including low-FODMAP fiber sources such as gluten-free grains, vegetables, and fruits, like berries, kiwi, and oranges, can help prevent constipation.
- Avoiding high-FODMAP foods that may trigger diarrhea: Some high-FODMAP foods, such as certain fruits, vegetables, and sweeteners, may trigger diarrhea in sensitive individuals. Avoiding or limiting the intake of these foods can help manage diarrhea.
- Monitoring portion sizes: Large portions of food, even if they are low in FODMAPs, can trigger digestive issues in some individuals. Monitoring portion sizes and eating moderate portions can help manage constipation and diarrhea.

Importance of Hydration and Fiber Intake

Hydration and fiber intake play a crucial role in maintaining digestive health on a low-FODMAP diet. Ensuring adequate water intake and incorporating low-FODMAP fiber sources into the diet can help prevent constipation and promote regular bowel movements.

The Role of Stress in Digestive Issues and Techniques for Managing Stress

Stress can exacerbate digestive issues such as bloating, gas, constipation, and diarrhea in some individuals. Stress triggers physiological responses in the body that can affect gut function. Here are some techniques for managing stress:

- Practicing relaxation techniques: Practices, like deep breathing, meditation, yoga, and other relaxation techniques, can be effective in managing stress and promoting relaxation of the muscles in the gut, potentially leading to relief from digestive discomfort.
- Regular exercise: It can help reduce stress and promote healthy digestion. Finding an exercise routine that works for an individual's fitness level and preferences can be beneficial for managing stress and digestive issues.
- Getting adequate sleep: Lack of sleep can contribute to stress and affect gut function. Prioritizing adequate sleep and establishing a regular sleep routine can help enhance digestive health and manage stress.

Gut-Healing Techniques

The gastrointestinal tract, commonly referred to as the gut, serves as a vital component of overall health and well-being. Its responsibilities include digestion, nutrient absorption, and waste elimination. Ensuring a well-maintained gut is crucial for optimal digestion, immune function, and overall wellness.

Gut-Healing Foods and Supplements

There are several foods and supplements that can support gut health and promote healing. These include:

- Bone broth: Bone broth is rich in nutrients such as collagen, amino acids, and minerals that can help repair and heal the gut lining and reduce inflammation.
- Ginger and turmeric: The anti-inflammatory properties of ginger and turmeric are renowned for their potential to alleviate gut inflammation and support the healing process.
- Glutamine: Glutamine is an amino acid that has been shown to support gut health by promoting the regeneration of gut lining cells and reducing inflammation.
- Omega-3 fatty acids: They are present in flaxseeds and fish have anti-inflammatory properties that can help reduce gut inflammation and promote gut healing.

Probiotics and Prebiotics

Probiotics are good and beneficial bacteria that can help restore the balance of gut microbiota, which is essential for gut health. Prebiotics are dietary fibers that act as food for probiotics, which help them thrive in the gut. Probiotics and prebiotics can be obtained from foods or supplements and can help improve gut health by promoting a healthy gut microbiome.

Other Natural Remedies for Digestive Issues

There are several other natural remedies that can support gut healing and help manage digestive issues. These include:

- Aloe vera: The anti-inflammatory properties of aloe vera make it a beneficial remedy for alleviating gut inflammation, supporting gut healing, and reducing digestive discomfort.
- Peppermint oil: Peppermint oil has been shown to have antispasmodic properties that can help relax gut muscles, reduce abdominal pain, and alleviate symptoms of irritable bowel syndrome (IBS).
- Slippery elm: Slippery elm is a herb that can help soothe irritated gut lining, reduce inflammation, and promote gut healing.
- DGL licorice: DGL (deglycyrrhizinated licorice) is a form of licorice that has been shown to have anti-inflammatory properties and can help soothe gut inflammation and promote healing.

Chapter 5:

THE MEAL PLANNING & 28-DAYS MEAL PLAN

Meal planning is a crucial aspect of successfully navigating the low-FODMAP diet, and a well-designed 28-day meal plan can be a game-changer. Imagine having delicious and satisfying meals ready to go without the stress of constantly searching for low-FODMAP recipes or figuring out what to eat. With a thoughtfully crafted meal plan, you can enjoy a variety of flavorful and nutritious low-FODMAP meals while ensuring you're meeting your dietary needs. From batch-cooked soups and stews to freezer-friendly casseroles and stir-fries, a 28-day meal plan can provide you with the tools to simplify your meal preparation, save time and effort, and ultimately identify your trigger foods with ease. Say goodbye to mealtime stress and hello to a well-organized and delicious low-FODMAP meal plan that will make your journey toward identifying your trigger foods a breeze.

High FODMAP Foods To Avoid

If you are trying a low-FODMAP diet or managing food intolerances related to FODMAPs, it's important to avoid or limit high-FODMAP foods. Here are some examples:

- Wheat and wheat products: This includes bread, pasta, cereals, and other foods made with wheat.
- Rye and rye products: This includes rye bread, rye crackers, and other foods made with rye.
- Barley and barley products: This includes barley bread, barley malt, and other foods made with barley.
- Certain fruits: Apples, pears, watermelon, cherries, mangoes, and nectarines are high in FODMAPs and should be limited or avoided.
- Certain vegetables: Onion, garlic, leeks, shallots, asparagus, artichokes, mushrooms, and cauliflower are high in FODMAPs and should be limited or avoided.
- Legumes: Lentils, beans, chickpeas, and other legumes are high in FODMAPs and may cause symptoms in some individuals.
- Dairy products: Milk, yogurt, ice cream, and soft cheeses are high in lactose, a type of FODMAP, and should be limited or avoided if you are lactose intolerant.

- Sweeteners: High fructose honey, agave syrup, corn syrup, and certain artificial sweeteners, like sorbitol, mannitol, and xylitol, are high in FODMAPs and should be avoided or limited.
- Certain beverages: Some alcoholic beverages, like beer and certain fruit juices, like apple or pear juice, are high in FODMAPs and should be limited or avoided.

Meal Planning

Planning and preparing meals during the elimination stage of a low-FODMAP diet can require some extra effort, but with some strategies in place, it is manageable. Here are some tips for meal planning and preparation:

Create a meal plan: Plan your meals ahead of time to ensure that you have a variety of low-FODMAP options available. Look for recipes and meal ideas that focus on whole, unprocessed foods such as meats, fish, eggs, vegetables, fruits, and grains, such as rice and quinoa, which are typically low in FODMAPs. Consider working with a registered dietitian who specializes in the low-FODMAP diet to help you make a well-balanced meal plan that specifically meets your nutritional requirements.

Batch cook: Batch cooking can save you time and effort during the elimination stage of this diet. Cook larger portions of low-FODMAP meals that can be divided into individual servings and stored in the refrigerator or freezer for later use. For example, you can cook a big pot of low-FODMAP soup, chili, or stew that can be portioned and frozen for future meals. This way, you'll have ready-made meals on hand when you're short on time or energy.

Freezer-friendly recipes: Look for freezer-friendly recipes that you can prepare in advance and store in the freezer for later use. Examples of freezer-friendly low-FODMAP meals include casseroles, stir-fries, and baked dishes, like lasagna or meatballs. These can be cooked, portioned, and stored in freezer-safe containers or bags for easy reheating and quick meals during busy times.

Easy-to-prepare meals and snacks: During the elimination stage of this diet, it's important to have some easy-to-prepare meals and snacks on hand for convenience. Some ideas include grilled or baked protein sources (such as chicken, fish, or tofu) with steamed or roasted low-FODMAP vegetables, simple stir-fries with low-FODMAP ingredients, or a sandwich made with gluten-free bread, low-FODMAP deli meat, and non-FODMAP fillings like lettuce, cucumber, and tomato. Snack options can include fresh fruits, hard-boiled eggs, lactose-free yogurt, or low-FODMAP nuts and seeds.

Stock low-FODMAP staples: Keep your pantry stocked with low-FODMAP staples to make meal preparation easier. Some examples include gluten-free grains like rice, quinoa, and oats; canned low-FODMAP beans like lentils and chickpeas; low-FODMAP broths or stocks; canned tomatoes; and low-FODMAP condiments like vinegar, mustard, and oils. Having these staples on hand can make it easier to whip up a quick and flavorful low-FODMAP meal.

Read labels carefully: When preparing meals during the elimination stage of this diet, it's important to read food labels carefully to avoid high-FODMAP ingredients. Look out for common FODMAPs such as wheat, garlic, onions, honey, high-fructose corn syrup, and lactose in food products. Choose products that are certified low-FODMAP or labeled as FODMAP-friendly whenever possible.

Experiment with low-FODMAP recipes: There are plenty of delicious low-FODMAP recipes available in this cookbook that can provide inspiration for your meal planning. Experiment with new recipes and try different low-FODMAP Ingredients to keep your meals interesting and flavorful during the elimination phase.

Low-FODMAP Foods To Enjoy

If you are following a low-FODMAP diet or managing food intolerances related to FODMAPs, there are several of delicious low-FODMAP foods that you can have. Here are some examples of low-FODMAP foods that you can include in your diet:

Proteins: Chicken, turkey, fish, eggs, tofu, tempeh, and lactose-free dairy items (lactose-free milk, hard cheeses and yogurt) are generally low in FODMAPs and can be included in your meals.

Carbohydrates: Rice (including white, brown, and basmati rice), quinoa, oats, gluten-free bread, corn-based products, and gluten-free pasta are typically well-tolerated on a low-FODMAP diet and can be used as carbohydrate sources.

Vegetables: Bell peppers, carrots, cucumbers, spinach, lettuce, zucchini, eggplant, and green beans are generally low in FODMAPs and can be included in your meals. It's important to note that some vegetables, such as broccoli, cabbage, and Brussels sprouts, may be high in FODMAPs in larger amounts and should be consumed in moderation.

Fruits: Strawberries, blueberries, raspberries, oranges, grapes, pineapple, and kiwi are generally low in FODMAPs and can be included in your diet. However, it's important to be considerate of portion sizes and avoid consuming large amounts of fruits that are higher in fructose, such as apples, pears, watermelon, and cherries.

Fats: Olive oil, avocado, coconut oil, and nuts (such as almonds, walnuts, and pecans) are generally low in FODMAPs and can be used as healthy fat sources in your meals.

Herbs and spices: Most of the herbs and spices are low in FODMAPs and can be used to add flavor to your meals without causing digestive discomfort.

Beverages: Water, herbal teas, black coffee (without added sweeteners), and lactose-free milk or milk alternatives (such as almond milk or coconut milk) are typically well-tolerated on a Low-FODMAP diet.

Reintroduction Phase

The reintroduction phase is an important step in the FODMAP diet, as it calls for systematically introducing the high-FODMAP foods back into your diet to determine your individual tolerance to these foods. The reintroduction phase typically occurs after a period of strict elimination of high-FODMAP foods, during which you have followed a low-FODMAP diet to alleviate the symptoms of food intolerances related to FODMAPs. The purpose of the reintroduction phase is to identify which specific FODMAPs or high- FODMAP foods trigger your symptoms and to determine your tolerance level for each of them. This can help you create a more personalized and sustainable long-term diet plan that includes a wider variety of foods while minimizing symptoms.

Start slowly: Begin by reintroducing one FODMAP group at a time. It's recommended to start with the group that you miss the most or suspect might be well-tolerated. For example, you could start with fructans, which are found in wheat, onions, and garlic.

Choose appropriate portion sizes: Start with a small portion size of the food you are reintroducing. For example, you could start with a small slice of bread or a small amount of onion or garlic.

Monitor symptoms: Keep a food and symptom diary to track how your body responds to the reintroduced FODMAPs. Note any changes in your symptoms, for instance bloating, gas, pain in the abdomen, or problems in bowel movements, over a 24-48 hour period, after consuming the reintroduced food.

Allow time for recovery: After reintroducing a FODMAP group, return to your low-FODMAP diet for a few days to allow your body to recover and stabilize before moving on to reintroduce another group.

Repeat the process: Continue to reintroduce one FODMAP group at a time, following the same process of starting with small portions, monitoring symptoms, and allowing time for recovery, until you have tested all the FODMAP groups that were previously restricted from your diet.

Interpret the results: Based on your food and symptom diary, you and your healthcare professional can review the results and determine which high-FODMAPs are well-tolerated and which may be trigger-foods for you. This information can help you customize your long-term diet plan to manage your symptoms effectively.

The reintroduction process can be complex, and it's important to do it under the guidance of a healthcare expert. They can provide personalized recommendations and ensure that you are reintroducing high-FODMAPs safely and effectively to identify your trigger foods and create a balanced and sustainable diet plan.

28-DAY MEAL PLAN

DAY 1	
Breakfast	Multi-Grain Bread
Lunch	Egg Salad
Dinner	Chicken Roulade
DAY 2	
Breakfast	Ricotta Pancakes
Lunch	Shrimp with Broccoli
Dinner	Chickpeas & Spinach Curry
DAY 3	
Breakfast	Veggie Frittata
Lunch	Salmon Burgers
Dinner	
DAY 4	
Breakfast	Acai Smoothie Bowl
Lunch	Veggie Lettuce Wraps
Dinner	Salmon & Quinoa Soup
DAY 5	
Breakfast	Salmon Omelet
Lunch	Orange & Beet Salad
Dinner	Ground Turkey with Green Beans
DAY 6	
Breakfast	Chia Seed Pudding
Lunch	Beef Burgers
Dinner	Lentil & Pumpkin Curry
DAY 7	
Breakfast	Banana Waffles
Lunch	Avocado & Bacon Soup
Dinner	Herbed Flank Steak
DAY 8	
Breakfast	Pineapple Smoothie
Lunch	Spiced Ground Chicken
Dinner	Seafood Combo
DAY 9	
Breakfast	Eggs with Beef & Tomatoes
Lunch	Stuffed Zucchini
Dinner	Herbed Flank Steak

DAY 10	
Breakfast	Blueberry Muffins
Lunch	Cucumber & Tomato Salad
Dinner	Ground Beef & Cabbage Soup

DAY 11	
Breakfast	Chia Seed Pudding
Lunch	Egg Drop Soup
Dinner	Lemony Chicken Breasts

DAY 12	
Breakfast	Ricotta Pancakes
Lunch	Chicken & Veggie Kabobs
Dinner	

DAY 13	
Breakfast	Yogurt & Cheese Bowl
Lunch	Shrimp with Broccoli
Dinner	Chicken Rolaude

DAY 14	
Breakfast	Spinach Smoothie
Lunch	Avocado Salad
Dinner	Turkey & Beans Chili

DAY 15	
Breakfast	Veggie Frittata
Lunch	Salmon Burgers
Dinner	Chickpeas & Spinach Curry

DAY 16	
Breakfast	French Toast
Lunch	Egg Drop Soup
Dinner	Beef with Bell Peppers

DAY 17	
Breakfast	Blueberry Oatmeal
Lunch	Turkey Meatloaf
Dinner	Parsley Pork Tenderloin

DAY 18	
Breakfast	Oat & Quinoa Granola
Lunch	Spinach with Cottage Cheese
Dinner	Pork Stew

DAY 19	
Breakfast	Eggs with Beef & Tomatoes
Lunch	Avocado & Bacon Soup
Dinner	Seafood Casserole

DAY 20	
Breakfast	Strawberry Smoothie
Lunch	Banana Curry
Dinner	Lemony Chicken Breasts

DAY 21	
Breakfast	Salmon Omelet
Lunch	Mixed Veggie Combo
Dinner	Dill Salmon

DAY 22	
Breakfast	Blueberry Muffins
Lunch	Turkey & Beans Meatballs
Dinner	Veggie Stew

DAY 23	
Breakfast	Acai Smoothie Bowl
Lunch	Stuffed Zucchini
Dinner	Parsley Pork Tenderloin

DAY 24	
Breakfast	Cheddar & Egg Scramble
Lunch	Spiced Ground Chicken
Dinner	Salmon & Quinoa Soup

DAY 25	
Breakfast	Multi-Grain Bread
Lunch	Beef Burgers
Dinner	Lentil & Pumpkin Curry

DAY 26	
Breakfast	Banana Waffles
Lunch	Spinach with Cottage Cheese
Dinner	Turkey & Beans Chili

DAY 27	
Breakfast	Buckwheat Porridge
Lunch	Turkey Meatloaf
Dinner	Dill Salmon

DAY 28	
Breakfast	Oat & Quinoa Granola
Lunch	Beef Stuffed Bell Peppers
Dinner	Veggie Stew

Chapter 6:
THE RECIPES

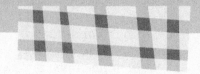

BREAKFAST RECIPES

LUNCH RECIPES

APPETIZER & SNACK RECIPES

MAIN DISH RECIPES

VEGETABLES & SALADS RECIPES

SIDE DISHES RECIPES

SMOOTHIES & DRINKS RECIPES

DESSERT RECIPES

KITCHEN STAPLE RECIPES

Low-FODMAP Acai Smoothie Bowl

Prep: 10 minutes
Total Time: 10 minutes
Serving portions: 2

Nutrition facts:
Calories 262, Total Fat 7.2 g, Saturated Fat 1.3 g, Cholesterol 0 mg, Sodium 146 mg, Total Carbs 40.1 g, Fiber 5 g, Sugar 20.8 g, Protein 12.3 g

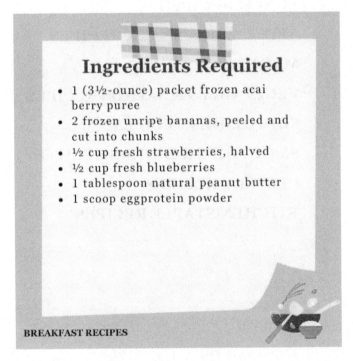

Ingredients Required

- 1 (3½-ounce) packet frozen acai berry puree
- 2 frozen unripe bananas, peeled and cut into chunks
- ½ cup fresh strawberries, halved
- ½ cup fresh blueberries
- 1 tablespoon natural peanut butter
- 1 scoop eggprotein powder

BREAKFAST RECIPES

Procedure of Cooking

1. In a high-power processor, put acai berry pureeand remaining ingredients. Process until perfectly smooth.
2. Immediately put the smoothie mixture into a bowl and enjoy.

Low-FODMAP Yogurt & Cottage Cheese Bowl

Prep: 10 minutes
Total Time: 10 minutes
Serving portions: 2

Nutrition facts:
Calories 244, Total Fat 16.2 g, Saturated Fat 5 g, Cholesterol 10 mg, Sodium 303 mg, Total Carbs 33.7 g, Fiber 6.7 g, Sugar 17.3 g, Protein 18.5 g

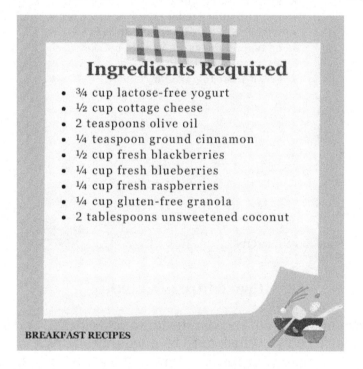

Ingredients Required

- ¾ cup lactose-free yogurt
- ½ cup cottage cheese
- 2 teaspoons olive oil
- ¼ teaspoon ground cinnamon
- ½ cup fresh blackberries
- ¼ cup fresh blueberries
- ¼ cup fresh raspberries
- ¼ cup gluten-free granola
- 2 tablespoons unsweetened coconut

BREAKFAST RECIPES

Procedure of Cooking

1. In a large-sized bowl, put in the yogurt, cheese, oil, and cinnamon. Blend thoroughly.
2. Divide the yogurt mixture into two serving bowls.
3. Top with berries, granola, and coconut. Enjoy!

Low-FODMAP Chia Seed Pudding

Prep: 10 minutes
Total Time: 10 minutes
Serving portions: 2

Nutrition facts:
Calories 103, Total Fat 8.4 g, Saturated Fat 0.7 g, Cholesterol 0 mg, Sodium 90 mg, Total Carbs 9.3 g, Fiber 7.2 g, Sugar 0.3 g, Protein 4.5 g

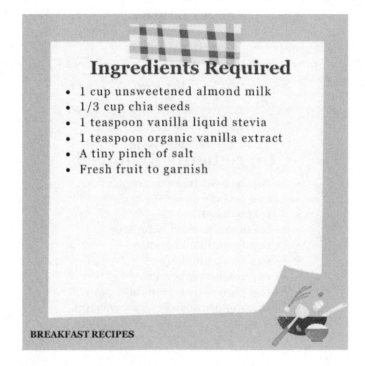

Ingredients Required

- 1 cup unsweetened almond milk
- 1/3 cup chia seeds
- 1 teaspoon vanilla liquid stevia
- 1 teaspoon organic vanilla extract
- A tiny pinch of salt
- Fresh fruit to garnish

BREAKFAST RECIPES

Procedure of Cooking

1. Place almond milk, chia seeds, stevia, vanilla extract, and salt in a medium-sized bowl. Whisk until blended thoroughly.
2. Put the mixture in your refrigerator for at least 10 minutes before enjoying it. Stir before eating. Garnish with your favorite fruit.

Low-FODMAP Blueberry Oatmeal

Prep: 10 minutes
Cook: 10 minutes
Total Time: 20 minutes
Serving portions: 2

Nutrition facts:
Calories 259, Total Fat 6.3 g, Saturated Fat 0.8 g, Cholesterol 0 mg, Sodium 186 mg,
Total Carbs 45.9 g, Fiber 5.6 g, Sugar 14.3 g, Protein 6.6 g

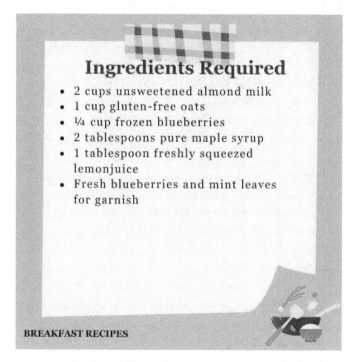

Ingredients Required

- 2 cups unsweetened almond milk
- 1 cup gluten-free oats
- ¼ cup frozen blueberries
- 2 tablespoons pure maple syrup
- 1 tablespoon freshly squeezed lemonjuice
- Fresh blueberries and mint leaves for garnish

BREAKFAST RECIPES

Procedure of Cooking

1. In a saucepan, put in the almond milkoats, and blueberries.
2. Cookat around medium heat for about 8-10 minutes.
3. Take the pan of oatmeal off of the burner. Blend in the maple syrup and lemonjuice.
4. Enjoy warm, garnishing with fresh blueberries and a mint leaf.

Low-FODMAP Buckwheat Porridge

Prep: 10 minutes
Cook: 17 minutes
Total Time: 27 minutes
Serving portions: 3

Nutrition facts:

Calories 145, Total Fat 2.3 g, Saturated Fat 0.3 g, Cholesterol 0 mg, Sodium 288 mg, Total Carbs 30.5 g, Fiber 3.2 g, Sugar 13.4 g, Protein 2.8 g

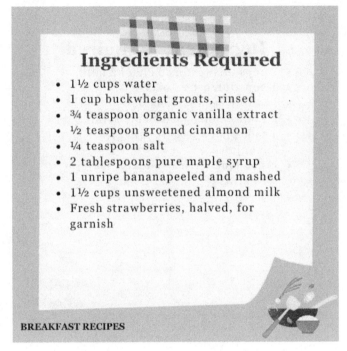

Ingredients Required

- 1½ cups water
- 1 cup buckwheat groats, rinsed
- ¾ teaspoon organic vanilla extract
- ½ teaspoon ground cinnamon
- ¼ teaspoon salt
- 2 tablespoons pure maple syrup
- 1 unripe bananapeeled and mashed
- 1½ cups unsweetened almond milk
- Fresh strawberries, halved, for garnish

BREAKFAST RECIPES

Procedure of Cooking

1. In a Dutch oven, put in the water, buckwheat, vanilla extractcinnamonand salton the burner at medium-high heat and cook until boiling.
2. Next, adjust the heat to medium-low and cook for 6 minutes, stirring from time to time.
3. Put in maple syrupbanana, and almond milk. Cook, covered, for 6 minutes.
4. Enjoy warm.

Low-FODMAP Cheddar & Egg Scramble

Prep: 10 minutes
Cook: 8 minutes
Total Time: 18 minutes
Serving portions: 6

Nutrition facts:
Calories 267, Total Fat 20.9 g, Saturated Fat 7.8 g, Cholesterol 392 mg,
Sodium 289 mg, Total Carbs 2.9 g, Fiber 0.7 g, Sugar 1.5 g, Protein 17.8 g

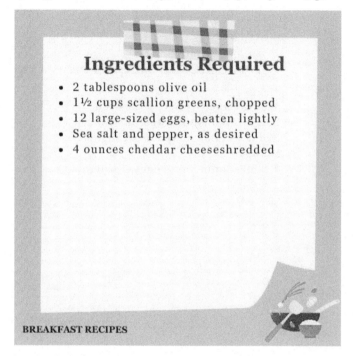

Ingredients Required

- 2 tablespoons olive oil
- 1½ cups scallion greens, chopped
- 12 large-sized eggs, beaten lightly
- Sea salt and pepper, as desired
- 4 ounces cheddar cheeseshredded

BREAKFAST RECIPES

Procedure of Cooking

1. Put oil in a large-sized, flat-bottomed wok. Put wok on the burner and sizzle at medium heat.
2. Add the scallion greens and cook for 4-5 minutes.
3. Put in the eggs, salt, and pepper. Cook for 3 minutes, stirring regularly.
4. Take off from burner and immediately mix in the cheese.
5. Enjoy immediately.

Low-FODMAP Salmon Omelet

Prep: 10 minutes
Cook: 5 minutes
Total Time: 15 minutes
Serving portions: 2

Nutrition facts:
Calories 309, Total Fat 24.9 g, Saturated Fat 11.8 g, Cholesterol 385 mg,
Sodium 406 mg, Total Carbs 1.1 g, Fiber 0 g, Sugar 1.1 g, Protein 20.8 g

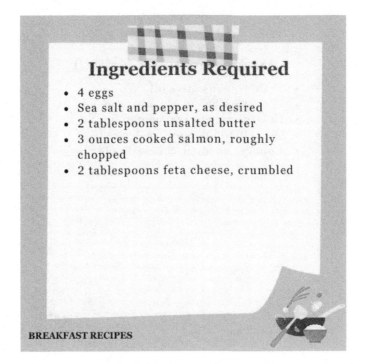

Ingredients Required

- 4 eggs
- Sea salt and pepper, as desired
- 2 tablespoons unsalted butter
- 3 ounces cooked salmon, roughly chopped
- 2 tablespoons feta cheese, crumbled

BREAKFAST RECIPES

Procedure of Cooking

1. In a bowl, put in the eggs, salt, and pepper. Gently stir until blended thoroughly.
2. In a frying pan, add the butter and let it melt on the burner at medium heat.
3. Place the beaten eggs into the pan evenly and cook for 1-2 minutes, without stirring.
4. Carefully lift the edges to allow the uncooked portion to flow underneath.
5. Place the salmon pieces into the center of the omelet and cook for 40-50 seconds.
6. Top with cheese and cook for 20-40 seconds.
7. Take off from burner and put the omelet onto a plate.
8. Enjoy immediately.

Low-FODMAP Eggs with Beef & Tomatoes

Prep: 15 minutes
Cook: 40 minutes
Total Time: 55 minutes
Serving portions: 4

Nutrition facts:
Calories 378, Total Fat 24.9 g, Saturated Fat 7.4 g, Cholesterol 229 mg,
Sodium 305 mg, Total Carbs 15.4 g, Fiber 5 g, Sugar 8.6 g, Protein 27.6 g

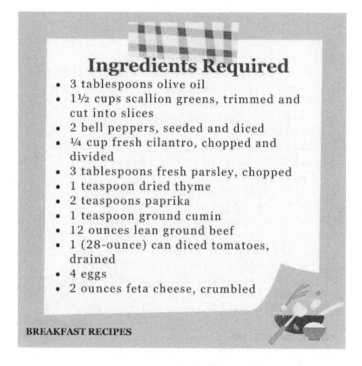

Ingredients Required

- 3 tablespoons olive oil
- 1½ cups scallion greens, trimmed and cut into slices
- 2 bell peppers, seeded and diced
- ¼ cup fresh cilantro, chopped and divided
- 3 tablespoons fresh parsley, chopped
- 1 teaspoon dried thyme
- 2 teaspoons paprika
- 1 teaspoon ground cumin
- 12 ounces lean ground beef
- 1 (28-ounce) can diced tomatoes, drained
- 4 eggs
- 2 ounces feta cheese, crumbled

BREAKFAST RECIPES

Procedure of Cooking

1. In a large-sized shallow flat-bottomed wok, put oil on the burner and sizzle at medium heat.
2. Add the scallion greens and cook for about 2-3 minutes.
3. Put in the bell peppers and cook for 5 minutes, stirring regularly.
4. Add 2 tablespoons of cilantro, parsley, thyme, paprika, and cumin. Cook for 2 minutes, stirring regularly.
5. Put in the ground beef and cook for about 4-5 minutes, stirring regularly.
6. Add the tomatoes, salt, and pepper. Cook for about 15-20 minutes, stirring from time to time.
7. With a spoon, make 4 wells in the cooked mixture.
8. Carefully crack 1 egg into each well and sprinkle each egg with a bit of salt.
9. Cover the wok and cook for about 5 minutes.
10. Take off from burner and enjoy hot, with the garnishing of remaining cilantro.

Low-FODMAP Vegetable Frittata

Prep: 15 minutes
Cook: 28 minutes
Total Time: 43 minutes
Serving portions: 8

Nutrition facts:
Calories 164, Total Fat 13.4 g, Saturated Fat 4 g, Cholesterol 173 mg, Sodium 226 mg, Total Carbs 4.2 g, Fiber 1.1 g, Sugar 2.2 g, Protein 8.1 g

Ingredients Required

- 1 small-sized zucchini, trimmed and cut into half-inch half moons
- 1 small-sized red bell pepper, seeded and diced
- 4 ounces broccoli, cut into small florets
- ½ cup scallion greens, chopped
- ¼ cup olive oil
- Sea salt and pepper, as desired
- 7 large eggs
- ¼ cup unsweetened almond milk
- 1/3 cup plus ¼ cup feta cheese, crumbled and divided
- 1/3 cup fresh parsley, finely chopped
- 1 teaspoon fresh thyme, stemmed and finely chopped
- ¼ teaspoon baking powder

BREAKFAST RECIPES

Procedure of Cooking

1. Preheat your oven to 450 °F.
2. Arrange a rack in the middle of oven.
3. While preheating, arrange a rimmed baking sheet in the oven to heat.
4. In a bowl, put in the zucchini, bell peppers, broccoli, scallion greens, 3 tablespoons of oil, salt, and pepper. Toss to blend.
5. Carefully take the hot baking sheet out of the oven.
6. Place the vegetable mixture onto the baking sheet and spread in an even layer.
7. Bake in your oven for about 15 minutes.
8. Take the baking sheet from oven and set it aside
9. Next set the temperature of oven to 400 °F.
10. In a bowl, put in the eggsalmond milk, 1/3 cup of feta, parsley, thyme, baking powder, salt, and pepper. Whisk until blended thoroughly.
11. Put in the roasted vegetables and stir to blend.
12. In a 10-inch cast-iron, flat-bottomed wok, heat the remaining oil at medium-high heat.
13. Place the egg mixture in the pan and spread in an even layer.
14. Cook for about 2-3 minutes.
15. Immediately put the cooking wok into the oven and bake the frittata in your oven for about 8-10 minutes.
16. Remove the cooking wok from oven and enjoy, garnished with the remaining feta.

Low-FODMAP Banana Waffles

Prep: 15 minutes
Cook: 20 minutes
Total Time: 35 minutes
Serving portions: 5

Nutrition facts:
Calories 360, Total Fat 29.8 g, Saturated Fat 4.3 g, Cholesterol 0 mg, Sodium 178 mg, Total Carbs 22.2 g, Fiber 8.8 g, Sugar 9.4 g, Protein 12.8 g

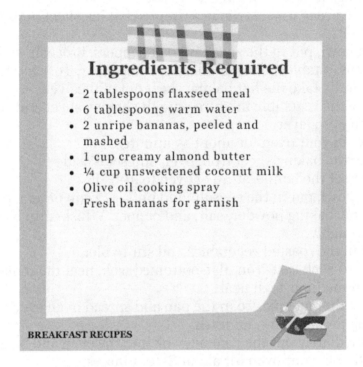

Ingredients Required

- 2 tablespoons flaxseed meal
- 6 tablespoons warm water
- 2 unripe bananas, peeled and mashed
- 1 cup creamy almond butter
- ¼ cup unsweetened coconut milk
- Olive oil cooking spray
- Fresh bananas for garnish

BREAKFAST RECIPES

Procedure of Cooking

1. In a small-sized bowl, put in flaxseed meal and warm water. Whisk until blended thoroughly.
2. Set it aside for about 10 minutes. In a medium-sized mixing bowl, put in the mashed bananas, almond butter, and coconut milk. Blend thoroughly.
3. Put in the flaxseed meal mixture and stir until blended thoroughly.
4. Preheat the waffle iron and lightly grease it with cooking spray.
5. Place desired amount of the waffle mixture in the preheated waffle iron. Cook for about 3-4 minutes.
6. Cook the the remaining waffles in the same method.
7. Enjoy warm, garnished with fresh banana disks.

Low-FODMAP Ricotta Pancakes

Prep: 10 minutes
Cook: 20 minutes
Total Time: 30 minutes
Serving portions: 4

Nutrition facts:
Calories 186, Total Fat 13.1 g, Saturated Fat 6.7 g, Cholesterol 202 mg,
Sodium 199 mg, Total Carbs 2.7 g, Fiber 0 g, Sugar 0.7 g, Protein 14.6 g

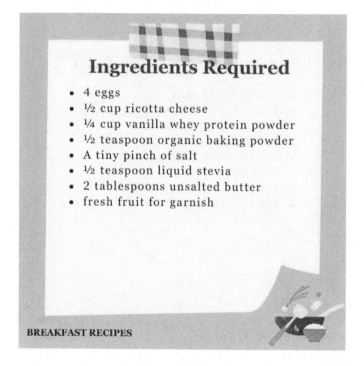

Ingredients Required

- 4 eggs
- ½ cup ricotta cheese
- ¼ cup vanilla whey protein powder
- ½ teaspoon organic baking powder
- A tiny pinch of salt
- ½ teaspoon liquid stevia
- 2 tablespoons unsalted butter
- fresh fruit for garnish

BREAKFAST RECIPES

Procedure of Cooking

1. In a clean food processor, put eggs and remaining ingredients. Process until blended thoroughly.
2. In a flat-bottomed wok, put in butter and let it melt on the burner at medium heat.
3. Put in the desired amount of the pancake mixture and spread it evenly.
4. Cook for about 2-3 minutes.
5. Flip and cook for about 1-2 minutes.
6. Cook the remaining pancakes in the same method.
7. Enjoy warm, garnished with fresh fruit.

Low-FODMAP French Toast

Prep: 10 minutes
Cook: 16 minutes
All the time: 26 minutes
Serving portions: 4

Nutrition facts:
Calories 130, Total Fat 7.9 g, Saturated Fat 1.4 g, Cholesterol 93 mg, Sodium 141 mg,
Total Carbs 10.2 g, Fiber 1.7 g, Sugar 0.3 g, Protein 4 g

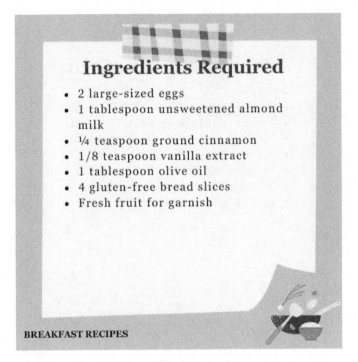

Ingredients Required

- 2 large-sized eggs
- 1 tablespoon unsweetened almond milk
- ¼ teaspoon ground cinnamon
- 1/8 teaspoon vanilla extract
- 1 tablespoon olive oil
- 4 gluten-free bread slices
- Fresh fruit for garnish

BREAKFAST RECIPES

Procedure of Cooking

1. In a medium-sized shallow bowl, put in milk, eggs, cinnamon, and vanilla extract. Whisk well.
2. In an anti-stick large-sized frying pan, put oil on the burner and sizzle at medium heat.
3. Dip bread slices in milk mixture and place into the pan.
4. Cook for about 2 minutes on each side.
5. Repeat with remaining bread slices.
6. Enjoy warm, with the garnishing of fresh fruit.

Low-FODMAP Blueberry Muffins

Prep: 15 minutes
Cook: 27 minutes
Total Time: 43 minutes
Serving portions: 8

Nutrition facts:
Calories 57, Total Fat 1.9 g, Saturated Fat 0.4 g, Cholesterol 20 mg, Sodium 88 mg,
Total Carbs 8 g, Fiber 1.7 g, Sugar 1.1 g, Protein 2.3 g

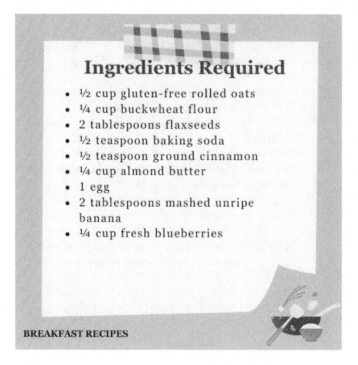

Ingredients Required

- ½ cup gluten-free rolled oats
- ¼ cup buckwheat flour
- 2 tablespoons flaxseeds
- ½ teaspoon baking soda
- ½ teaspoon ground cinnamon
- ¼ cup almond butter
- 1 egg
- 2 tablespoons mashed unripe banana
- ¼ cup fresh blueberries

BREAKFAST RECIPES

Procedure of Cooking

1. Preheat your oven to 375 °F.
2. Lightly grease 8 holes of a muffin pan.
3. In a clean blender, place oats and remaining ingredients, except the blueberries, and process until perfectly smooth and creamy.
4. Place the blended mixture into a bowl and fold in blueberries.
5. Spoon the blended mixture into the muffin holes evenly.
6. Bake in your oven for 10-12 minutes.
7. Take the muffin tin out of the oven and place onto a metal rack to cool for almost 10 minutes.
8. Invert the muffins onto the metal rack to cool before enjoying.

Low-FODMAP Multi-Grain Bread

Prep: 15 minutes
Cook: 50 minutes
Total Time: 1 hour 5 minutes
Serving portions: 14

Nutrition facts:
Calories 180, Total Fat 4.9 g, Saturated Fat 3.4 g, Cholesterol 0 mg, Sodium 259 mg,
Total Carbs 32.5 g, Fiber 11.1 g, Sugar 2.6 g, Protein 3.2 g

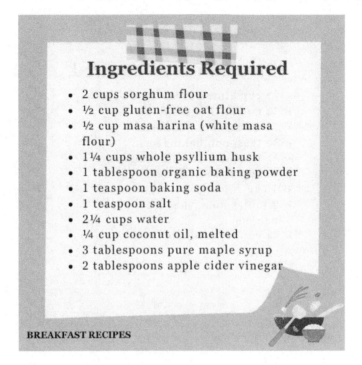

Ingredients Required

- 2 cups sorghum flour
- ½ cup gluten-free oat flour
- ½ cup masa harina (white masa flour)
- 1¼ cups whole psyllium husk
- 1 tablespoon organic baking powder
- 1 teaspoon baking soda
- 1 teaspoon salt
- 2¼ cups water
- ¼ cup coconut oil, melted
- 3 tablespoons pure maple syrup
- 2 tablespoons apple cider vinegar

BREAKFAST RECIPES

Procedure of Cooking

1. Preheat your oven to 375 °F.
2. Grease a loaf pan. (loaf pan standard size)
3. In a large-sized bowl, blend together the flours, psyllium husk, baking powder, baking soda, and salt.
4. In another bowl, put in water, coconut oil, maple syrup, and vinegar. Whisk until blended thoroughly.
5. Add the oil mixture into the bowl of flour mixture. Stir until just blended.
6. Place the blended mixture into the loaf pan.
7. Bake it in your oven for about 50-60 minutes.
8. Remove the loaf pan from oven and place onto a metal rack to cool for 10 minutes.
9. Carefully turn the bread onto the metal rack to cool thoroughly before slicing.
10. Cut the bread loaf into desired-sized slices and enjoy.

Low-FODMAP Oats & Quinoa Granola

Prep: 10 minutes
Cook: 30 minutes
Total Time: 40 minutes
Serving portions: 12

Nutrition facts:
Calories 168, Total Fat 9.2 g, Saturated Fat 1.4 g, Cholesterol 0 mg, Sodium 24 mg,
Total Carbs 56.6 g, Fiber 5 g, Sugar 3.4 g, Protein 4.5 g

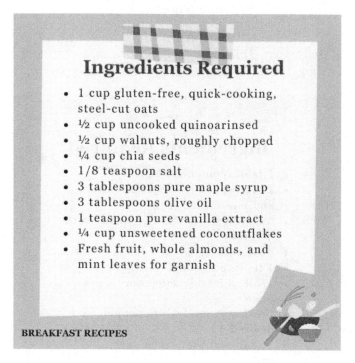

Ingredients Required

- 1 cup gluten-free, quick-cooking, steel-cut oats
- ½ cup uncooked quinoarinsed
- ½ cup walnuts, roughly chopped
- ¼ cup chia seeds
- 1/8 teaspoon salt
- 3 tablespoons pure maple syrup
- 3 tablespoons olive oil
- 1 teaspoon pure vanilla extract
- ¼ cup unsweetened coconutflakes
- Fresh fruit, whole almonds, and mint leaves for garnish

BREAKFAST RECIPES

Procedure of Cooking

1. Preheat your oven to 325 °F.
2. Arrange a rack on a slot from the bottom of oven.
3. Arrange baking paper to cover a large-sized baking sheet.
4. In a medium-sized bowl, put in oatsquinoawalnuts, chia seeds and salt
5. Add maple syrup, oil, and vanilla extract. Blend thoroughly.
6. Put the oat mixture onto the baking sheet and spread in an even layer.
7. Bake in your oven for 25 minutes.
8. Sprinkle the top of the granola with coconut flakes and bake the granola in your oven for 5 minutes more.
9. Take out of the oven and set it aside to cool thoroughly.
10. Break the granola into pieces and enjoy with your favorite milk and toppings, or alone as a snack.

LUNCH RECIPES

Low-FODMAP Egg Drop Soup

Prep: 10 minutes
Cook: 20 minutes
Total Time: 30 minutes
Serving portions: 6

Nutrition facts:
Calories 92, Net Carbs 3.2 g, Total Fat 5.3 g, Saturated Fat 1.3 g, Cholesterol 55 mg, Sodium 787 mg, Total Carbs 3.4 g, Fiber 0.2 g, Sugar 1.2 g, Protein 7 g

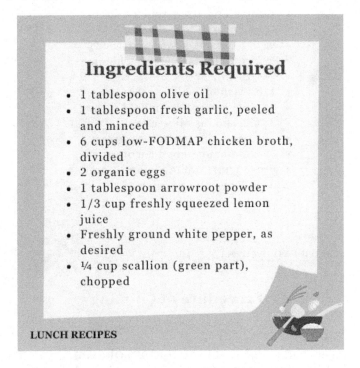

Ingredients Required

- 1 tablespoon olive oil
- 1 tablespoon fresh garlic, peeled and minced
- 6 cups low-FODMAP chicken broth, divided
- 2 organic eggs
- 1 tablespoon arrowroot powder
- 1/3 cup freshly squeezed lemon juice
- Freshly ground white pepper, as desired
- ¼ cup scallion (green part), chopped

Procedure of Cooking

1. In a large-sized soup pan, put oil on the burner and sizzle at medium-high heat.
2. Cook garlic for 1 minute.
3. Add 5½ cups of broth and cook until boiling at high heat.
4. Adjust the heat to medium and cook for about 5 minutes.
5. Meanwhile, in a bowl, add in eggs, arrowroot powder, lemon juice, white pepper, and remaining broth. Beat until blended thoroughly.
6. Slowly, pour in egg mixture into the pan, stirring constantly.
7. Simmer for about 5-6 minutes, stirring regularly.
8. Enjoy hot, with the garnishing of scallions.

Low-FODMAP Avocado & Bacon Soup

Prep: 15 minutes
Cook: 8 minutes
Total Time: 23 minutes
Serving portions: 4

Nutrition facts:
Calories 520, Net Carbs 3.2 g, Total Fat 41.7 g, Saturated Fat 11.7 g, Cholesterol 62 mg, Sodium 2000 mg, Total Carbs 9 g, Fiber 5.8 g, Sugar 1.1 g, Protein 27.5 g

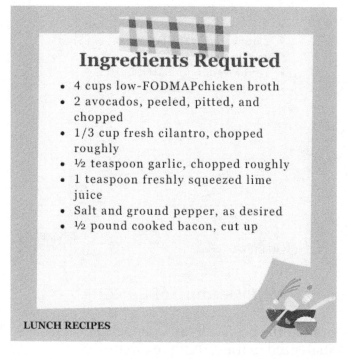

Ingredients Required

- 4 cups low-FODMAP chicken broth
- 2 avocados, peeled, pitted, and chopped
- 1/3 cup fresh cilantro, chopped roughly
- ½ teaspoon garlic, chopped roughly
- 1 teaspoon freshly squeezed lime juice
- Salt and ground pepper, as desired
- ½ pound cooked bacon, cut up

LUNCH RECIPES

Procedure of Cooking

1. In a large-sized saucepan, put the broth on the burner at medium-high heat and cook until boiling.
2. Adjust the heat to low.
3. Into a clean processor, put the avocadoes, cilantro, garlic, and lime juice. Process until finely blended.
4. Add 1 cup of the chicken broth and process until perfectly smooth.
5. Put the avocado mixture into the pan of remaining simmering broth and stir to blend.
6. Blend in the salt and pepper and cook for about 2-3 minutes.
7. Top with bacon pieces and enjoy immediately.

Low-FODMAP Beef Burgers

Prep: 10 minutes
Cook: 8 minutes
Total Time: 18 minutes
Serving portions: 2

Nutrition facts:
Calories 260, Total Fat 16.5 g, Saturated Fat 8.2 g, Cholesterol 94 mg,
Sodium 313 mg, Total Carbs 1.6 g, Fiber 0.7 g, Sugar 0.1 g, Protein 27.2 g

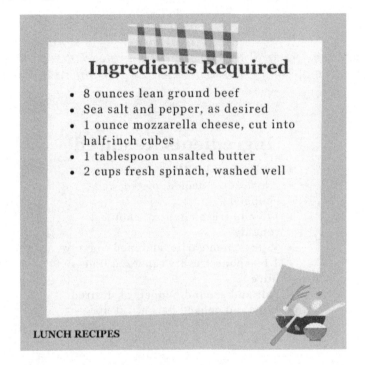

Ingredients Required

- 8 ounces lean ground beef
- Sea salt and pepper, as desired
- 1 ounce mozzarella cheese, cut into half-inch cubes
- 1 tablespoon unsalted butter
- 2 cups fresh spinach, washed well

LUNCH RECIPES

Procedure of Cooking

1. In a bowl, put in the beef, salt, and pepper. Stir until blended thoroughly.
2. Make 2 equal-sized patties from the mixture.
3. Place a mozzarella cube inside of each patty and surround it with the beef.
4. In a frying pan, put in butter and let it melt on the burner at medium heat.
5. Cook the patties for about 3-4 minutes on each side.
6. Divide the spinach onto serving plates and top each with 1 patty.
7. Enjoy immediately.

Low-FODMAP Turkey & Beans Meatballs

Prep: 15 minutes
Cook: 12 minutes
Total Time: 27 minutes
Serving portions: 8

Nutrition facts:
Calories 291, Total Fat 13 g, Saturated Fat 2 g, Cholesterol 58 mg, Sodium 113 mg,
Total Carbs 24.6 g, Fiber 5.2 g, Sugar 2 g, Protein 23.2 g

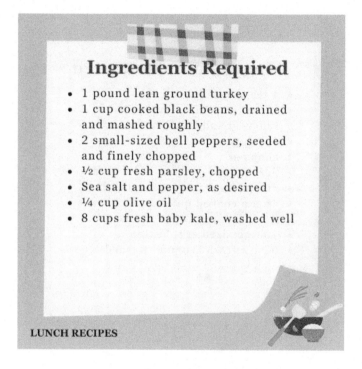

Ingredients Required

- 1 pound lean ground turkey
- 1 cup cooked black beans, drained and mashed roughly
- 2 small-sized bell peppers, seeded and finely chopped
- ½ cup fresh parsley, chopped
- Sea salt and pepper, as desired
- ¼ cup olive oil
- 8 cups fresh baby kale, washed well

LUNCH RECIPES

Procedure of Cooking

1. In a large-sized bowl, put in ground turkey and remaining ingredients, except for the oil, and blend until blended thoroughly.
2. Make equal-sized balls from the mixture.
3. In a large-sized, anti-sticking, flat-bottomed wok, put oil on the burner and sizzle at medium heat.
4. Cook meatballs for about 5-7 minutes, uncovered
5. Cover the wok and cook for about 5 minutes more.
6. Enjoy hot alongside the kale.

Low-FODMAP Salmon Burgers

Prep: 15 minutes
Cook: 15 minutes
Total Time: 30 minutes
Serving portions: 5

Nutrition facts:
Calories 289, Total Fat 13.2 g, Saturated Fat 2.5 g, Cholesterol 89 mg,
Sodium 189 mg, Total Carbs 19.2 g, Fiber 3.4 g, Sugar 3.1 g, Protein 23.7 g

Ingredients Required

- 1 teaspoon olive oil
- 1 cup fresh kale, tough ribs removed and chopped
- 1/3 cup scallion greens, finely chopped
- Sea salt and pepper, as desired
- 16 ounces skinless salmon fillets
- ¾ cup cooked quinoa
- 2 tablespoons Dijon mustard
- 1 large-sized egg, beaten
- 5 cups fresh arugula, washed
- 2 cups grape tomatoes, halved

LUNCH RECIPES

Procedure of Cooking

1. For burgers: in a large-sized anti-sticking, flat-bottomed wok, put oil on the burner and sizzle at medium heat.
2. Cook the kalescallion greens, salt, and pepper for about 4-5 minutes.
3. Take off from burner and put the kale mixture into a large-sized bowl.
4. Set it aside to cool slightly.
5. With a fork, shred 4 ounces of salmon and put it into the bowl of kale mixture.
6. Into a clean food processor, put the remaining salmon and process until finely chopped.
7. Put the processed salmon into the bowl of kale mixture.
8. Next, put in remaining ingredients, except for arugula and tomatoes, and stir until fully blended.
9. Make 5 equal-sized patties from the mixture.
10. Put a lightly greased anti-sticking, flat-bottomed wok on the burner and sizzle at medium heat.
11. Cook patties for about 4-5 minutes on each side.
12. Serve immediately alongside a salad of arugula and tomatoes.

Low-FODMAP Beef-Stuffed Bell Peppers

Prep: 15 minutes
Cook: 20 minutes
Total Time: 35 minutes
Serving portions: 4

Nutrition facts:
Calories 264, Total Fat 16.3 g, Saturated Fat 9.4 g, Cholesterol 52 mg,
Sodium 259 mg, Total Carbs 15.5 g, Fiber 3.4 g, Sugar 8.8 g, Protein 16.5 g

Ingredients Required

- 2 teaspoons coconut oil
- 1 pound lean ground beef
- 1 cup fresh oyster mushrooms, chopped
- 1½ cups scallion greens, chopped
- Sea salt and pepper, as desired
- ½ cup tomato puree
- 4 large bell peppers, halved lengthwise and cored
- 1 cup water
- 4 ounces sharp cheddar cheese, shredded

LUNCH RECIPES

Procedure of Cooking

1. Melt the coconut oil in a flat-bottomed wok at medium-high heat.
2. Add beef and cook for about 5 minutes, crumbling with the spoon.
3. Add in the mushrooms and scallion greens. Cook for about 5-6 minutes.
4. Put in salt and pepper. Cook for almost 1 minute
5. Take the pan of beef mixture from burner and drain off the excess grease.
6. Add in the tomato puree and stir to blend.
7. Meanwhile, in a large-sized microwave-safe dish, arrange the bell peppers, cut-side down.
8. Pour the water in the baking dish.
9. With plastic wrap, cover the baking dish and microwave on high for about 4-5 minutes.
10. Take out of microwave and uncover the baking dish.
11. Drain the water completely.
12. Next, in the baking dish, arrange the bell peppers, cut-side up.
13. Stuff the bell peppers evenly with beef mixture and top with cheese.
14. Microwave on high for about 2-3 minutes.
15. Enjoy warm.

Low-FODMAP Turkey Meatloaf

Prep: 15 minutes
Cook: 40 minutes
Total Time: 55 minutes
Serving portions: 10

Nutrition facts:
Calories 224, Total Fat 12.7 g, Saturated Fat 5.8 g, Cholesterol 99 mg,
Sodium 325 mg, Total Carbs 4.6 g, Fiber 0.2 g, Sugar 3.1 g, Protein 22.7 g

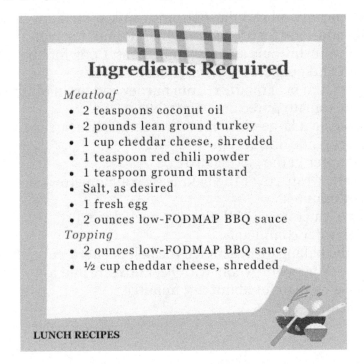

Ingredients Required

Meatloaf
- 2 teaspoons coconut oil
- 2 pounds lean ground turkey
- 1 cup cheddar cheese, shredded
- 1 teaspoon red chili powder
- 1 teaspoon ground mustard
- Salt, as desired
- 1 fresh egg
- 2 ounces low-FODMAP BBQ sauce

Topping
- 2 ounces low-FODMAP BBQ sauce
- ½ cup cheddar cheese, shredded

LUNCH RECIPES

Procedure of Cooking

1. Preheat your oven to 400 °F.
2. Grease a 9x13-inch casserole dish with cooking spray.
3. For meatloaf: add all of the ground turkey and remaining meatloaf ingredients into a bowl and stir until blended thoroughly.
4. Place the mixture into the casserole dish evenly and press to smooth the surface.
5. Coat the top of meatloaf with BBQ sauce evenly and sprinkle with the cheese.
6. Bake it in your oven for 40 minutes.
7. Take the meatloaf out of the oven and place onto a metal rack to cool slightly.
8. Cut the meatloaf into desired-sized slices and enjoy warm.

Low-FODMAP Chicken & Vegetable Kabobs

Prep: 15 minutes
Cook: 8 minutes
Total Time: 23 minutes
Serving portions: 6

Nutrition facts:
Calories 201, Net Carbs 3.2 g, Total Fat 10.6 g, Saturated Fat 1.7 g, Cholesterol 63 mg,
Sodium 99 mg, Total Carbs 4.3 g, Fiber 1.1 g, Sugar 2.6 g, Protein 22.3 g

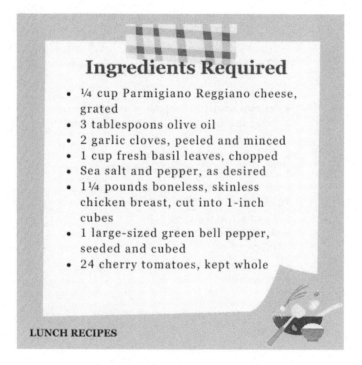

Ingredients Required

- ¼ cup Parmigiano Reggiano cheese, grated
- 3 tablespoons olive oil
- 2 garlic cloves, peeled and minced
- 1 cup fresh basil leaves, chopped
- Sea salt and pepper, as desired
- 1¼ pounds boneless, skinless chicken breast, cut into 1-inch cubes
- 1 large-sized green bell pepper, seeded and cubed
- 24 cherry tomatoes, kept whole

LUNCH RECIPES

Procedure of Cooking

1. Add cheese, butter, garlic, basil, salt, and pepper into a clean food processor and process until perfectly smooth.
2. Put this basil mixture into a large-sized bowl.
3. Add the chicken cubes and blend thoroughly.
4. Cover the bowl and put in your refrigerator to marinate for at least 4-5 hours.
5. Preheat the grill to medium-high heat. Generously, grease the grill grate.
6. Thread the chicken, bell pepper cubes, and whole tomatoes onto presoaked wooden skewers.
7. Place the skewers onto the grill and cook for about 6-8 minutes, flipping from time to time.
8. Remove skewers from the grill and place onto a platter to rest for 5 minutes before enjoying them.

Low-FODMAP Spiced Ground Chicken

Prep: 10 minutes
Cook: 11 minutes
Total Time: 21 minutes
Serving portions: 4

Nutrition facts:
Calories 293, Total Fat 17.2 g, Saturated Fat 4.2 g, Cholesterol 88 mg,
Sodium 129 mg, Total Carbs 1.4 g, Fiber 0.4 g, Sugar 0.4 g, Protein 30.4 g

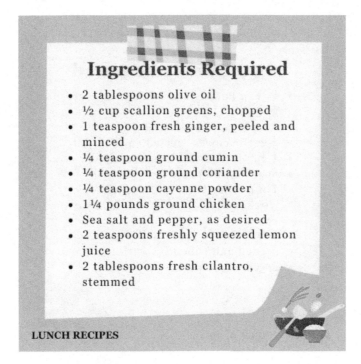

Ingredients Required

- 2 tablespoons olive oil
- ½ cup scallion greens, chopped
- 1 teaspoon fresh ginger, peeled and minced
- ¼ teaspoon ground cumin
- ¼ teaspoon ground coriander
- ¼ teaspoon cayenne powder
- 1¼ pounds ground chicken
- Sea salt and pepper, as desired
- 2 teaspoons freshly squeezed lemon juice
- 2 tablespoons fresh cilantro, stemmed

LUNCH RECIPES

Procedure of Cooking

1. In a flat-bottomed wok, put oil on the burner and sizzle at medium heat.
2. Cook the scallion greens, ginger, and spices for about 2-3 minutes.
3. Put in the ground chicken, salt, and pepper. Cook for about 6-7 minutes, breaking up the meat into smaller pieces with a wooden spoon.
4. Add lemon juice and cilantro. Cook for 1 minute.
5. Enjoy hot.

Low-FODMAP Shrimp with Broccoli

Prep: 15 minutes
Cook: 8 minutes
Total Time: 23 minutes
Serving portions: 6

Nutrition facts:
Calories 204, Total Fat 8.7 g, Saturated Fat 1 g, Cholesterol 223 mg, Sodium 722 mg, Total Carbs 7 g, Fiber 2.1 g, Sugar 2.5 g, Protein 27 g

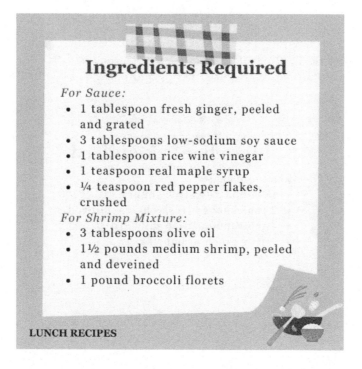

Ingredients Required

For Sauce:
- 1 tablespoon fresh ginger, peeled and grated
- 3 tablespoons low-sodium soy sauce
- 1 tablespoon rice wine vinegar
- 1 teaspoon real maple syrup
- ¼ teaspoon red pepper flakes, crushed

For Shrimp Mixture:
- 3 tablespoons olive oil
- 1½ pounds medium shrimp, peeled and deveined
- 1 pound broccoli florets

LUNCH RECIPES

Procedure of Cooking

1. For sauce: in a bowl, place ginger and remaining sauce ingredients. Whisk until blended thoroughly. Set it aside.
2. In a large-sized, flat-bottomed wok, put oil on the burner and sizzle at medium-high heat.
3. Cook shrimp for 2 minutes, stirring from time to time.
4. Put in the broccoli and cook for about 3-4 minutes, stirring regularly.
5. Add in the sauce mixture and cook for about 1-2 minutes.
6. Enjoy immediately.

APPETIZER & SNACK RECIPES

Low-FODMAP Deviled Eggs

Prep: 15 minutes
Cook: 5 minutes
Total Time: 20 minutes
Serving portions: 6

Nutrition facts:
Calories 81, Total Fat 5.2 g, Saturated Fat 1.7 g, Cholesterol 187 mg, Sodium 107 mg, Total Carbs 1.3 g, Fiber 0.1 g, Sugar 1.2 g, Protein 7 g

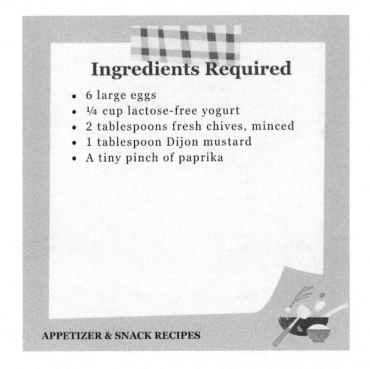

Ingredients Required

- 6 large eggs
- ¼ cup lactose-free yogurt
- 2 tablespoons fresh chives, minced
- 1 tablespoon Dijon mustard
- A tiny pinch of paprika

APPETIZER & SNACK RECIPES

Procedure of Cooking

1. In a saucepan of water, put in the eggs on the burner at high heat and cook until boiling.
2. Cover the pan of eggs and immediately take off from burner.
3. Set the pan of eggs aside, covered for at least 10-15 minutes.
4. Drain the eggs and let them cool completely.
5. Peel the eggs and, with a sharp knife, slice them in half.
6. Take the yolks out of egg halves.
7. Carefully scoop out the yolks from each egg half.
8. In a clean processor, put the egg yolks and yogurt and process until perfectly smooth.
9. Put the yogurt mixture into a bowl.
10. Put in the scallion greens, chives, and mustard. Stir to blend.
11. Spoon the yogurt mixture into each egg half evenly.
12. Serve with a sprinkling of paprika.

Low-FODMAP Stuffed Cherry Tomatoes

Prep: 20 minutes
Total Time: 20 minutes
Serving portions: 12

Nutrition facts:
Calories 80, Total Fat 3.8 g, Saturated Fat 1.8 g, Cholesterol 8 mg, Sodium 51 mg, Total Carbs 10.6 g, Fiber 3 g, Sugar 6.7 g, Protein 2.8 g

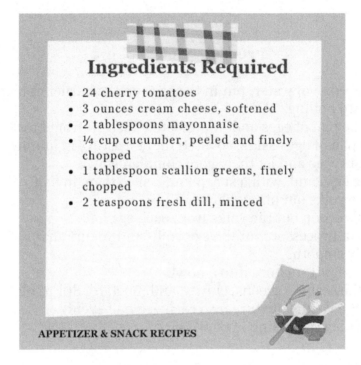

Ingredients Required

- 24 cherry tomatoes
- 3 ounces cream cheese, softened
- 2 tablespoons mayonnaise
- ¼ cup cucumber, peeled and finely chopped
- 1 tablespoon scallion greens, finely chopped
- 2 teaspoons fresh dill, minced

APPETIZER & SNACK RECIPES

Procedure of Cooking

1. Carefully cut a thin slice from the top of each cherry tomato.
2. With the tip of a knife, carefully the remove the pulp of each cherry tomato and discard it.
3. Arrange the tomatoes onto paper towels to drain, cut side down.
4. Place the cream cheese and mayonnaise in a bowl and whisk until smooth.
5. Put in the cucumber, scallion greens, and dill. Stir to blend.
6. With a spoon, place the cheese mixture into each tomato.
7. Arrange the tomatoes onto a platter and put in your refrigerator to chill slightly before enjoying them.

Low-FODMAP Popcorn Chicken

Prep: 15 minutes
Cook: 25 minutes
Total Time: 40 minutes
Serving portions: 3

Nutrition facts:
Calories 290, Total Fat 21.4 g, Saturated Fat 16.2 g, Cholesterol 50 mg,
Sodium 107 mg, Total Carbs 7.7 g, Fiber 2.9 g, Sugar 3.6 g, Protein 18.2 g

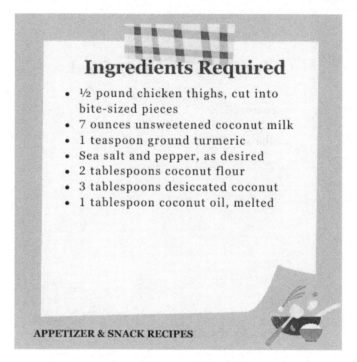

Ingredients Required

- ½ pound chicken thighs, cut into bite-sized pieces
- 7 ounces unsweetened coconut milk
- 1 teaspoon ground turmeric
- Sea salt and pepper, as desired
- 2 tablespoons coconut flour
- 3 tablespoons desiccated coconut
- 1 tablespoon coconut oil, melted

APPETIZER & SNACK RECIPES

Procedure of Cooking

1. In a large-sized bowl, stir together chicken, coconut milk, turmeric, salt, and pepper.
2. Cover and put in your refrigerator to marinate overnight.
3. Preheat the oven to 390°F.
4. In a shallow dish, blend together coconut flour and desiccated coconut.
5. Coat the chicken pieces in coconut mixture evenly.
6. Arrange chicken pieces onto a baking sheet and drizzle with oil evenly.
7. Bake in your oven for about 20-25 minutes. Enjoy!

Low-FODMAP Bacon-Wrapped Scallops

Prep: 15 minutes
Cook: 15 minutes
All the time: 30 minutes
Serving portions: 9

Nutrition facts:
Calories 103, Total Fat 5.6 g, Saturated Fat 1.2 g, Cholesterol 24 mg, Sodium 187 mg,
Total Carbs 1.4 g, Fiber 0 g, Sugar 0 g, Protein 11.5 g

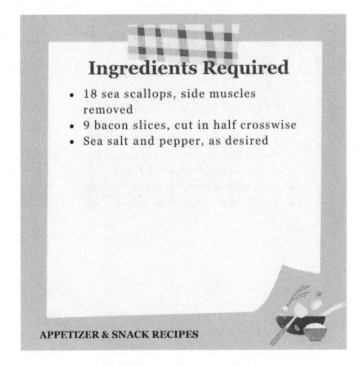

Ingredients Required

- 18 sea scallops, side muscles removed
- 9 bacon slices, cut in half crosswise
- Sea salt and pepper, as desired

APPETIZER & SNACK RECIPES

Procedure of Cooking

1. Preheat your oven to 425 °F.
2. Arrange baking paper to cover a large-sized baking sheet.
3. Wrap each scallop with 1 bacon slice half and secure with toothpick.
4. Drizzle the scallops with oil evenly and then season with salt and pepper.
5. Arrange scallops onto the baking sheet.
6. Bake them in your oven for about 12-15 minutes.
7. Take the baking sheet of scallops from oven and enjoy immediately.

Low-FODMAP Coconut Shrimp

Prep: 15 minutes
Cook: 20 minutes
Total Time: 35 minutes
Serving portions: 8

Nutrition facts:
Calories 120, Total Fat 4.1 g, Saturated Fat 2.1 g, Cholesterol 18 mg, Sodium 190 mg, Total Carbs 4.6 g, Fiber 0.6 g, Sugar 1 g, Protein 15.5 g

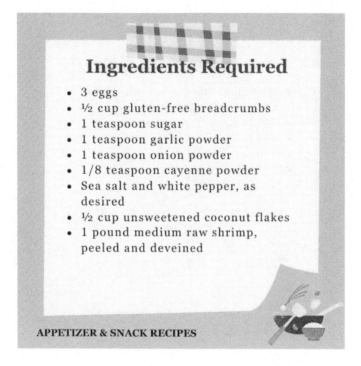

Ingredients Required

- 3 eggs
- ½ cup gluten-free breadcrumbs
- 1 teaspoon sugar
- 1 teaspoon garlic powder
- 1 teaspoon onion powder
- 1/8 teaspoon cayenne powder
- Sea salt and white pepper, as desired
- ½ cup unsweetened coconut flakes
- 1 pound medium raw shrimp, peeled and deveined

APPETIZER & SNACK RECIPES

Procedure of Cooking

1. Preheat the oven to 425 °F.
2. Arrange a baking paper to cover a large-sized baking sheet.
3. In a shallow dish, crack the eggs and beat lightly.
4. In a second shallow dish, blend together the remaining ingredients, except coconut and shrimp.
5. In a third shallow dish, place the coconut flakes.
6. First, dip the shrimp in the eggs and then roll it into breadcrumbs mixture.
7. Again, dip in eggs and then roll into coconut flakes.
8. Place the shrimp onto the baking sheet.
9. Bake in your oven for about 15-20 minutes.
10. Enjoy warm.

Low-FODMAP Zucchini Chips

Prep: 10 minutes
Cook: 15 minutes
Total time: 25 minutes
Serving portions: 2

Nutrition facts:
Calories 57, Total Fat 4.9 g, Saturated Fat 0.7 g, Cholesterol 0 mg, Sodium 88 mg, Total Carbs 3.4 g, Fiber 1.1 g, Sugar 1.7 g, Protein 1.2 g

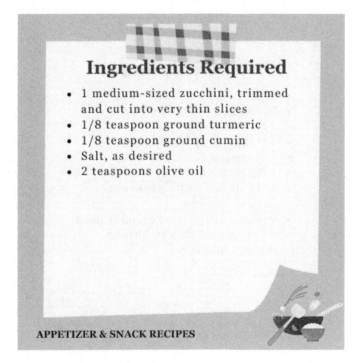

Ingredients Required

- 1 medium-sized zucchini, trimmed and cut into very thin slices
- 1/8 teaspoon ground turmeric
- 1/8 teaspoon ground cumin
- Salt, as desired
- 2 teaspoons olive oil

APPETIZER & SNACK RECIPES

Procedure of Cooking

1. Preheat your oven to 400 °F.
2. Arrange baking papers to cover two large-sized baking sheets.
3. In a large-sized bowl, put in zucchini slices, spices, salt, and oil. Toss to blend.
4. Put the zucchini onto the baking sheets.
5. Bake them in your oven for about 10-15 minutes, until crisp.
6. Enjoy immediately.

Low-FODMAP Potato Sticks

Prep: 10 minutes
Cook: 15 minutes
Total Time: 25 minutes
Serving portions: 2

Nutrition facts:
Calories 204, Total Fat 7.3 g, Saturated Fat 1.1 g, Cholesterol 0 mg, Sodium 92 mg,
Total Carbs 32.6 g, Fiber 4.2 g, Sugar 1.5 g, Protein 3.8 g

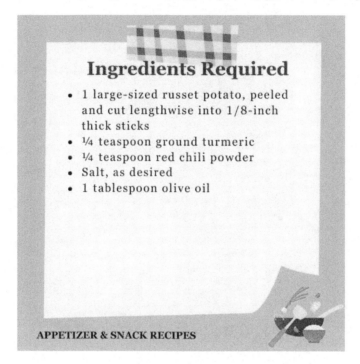

Ingredients Required

- 1 large-sized russet potato, peeled and cut lengthwise into 1/8-inch thick sticks
- ¼ teaspoon ground turmeric
- ¼ teaspoon red chili powder
- Salt, as desired
- 1 tablespoon olive oil

APPETIZER & SNACK RECIPES

Procedure of Cooking

1. Preheat your oven to 400 °F.
2. Arrange baking papers onto two large-sized baking sheets.
3. In a large-sized bowl, put in potato sticks, spices, salt, and oil. Toss to blend.
4. Place the potato sticks onto the baking sheets and arrange in one layer.
5. Bake in your oven for about 10 minutes.
6. Enjoy immediately.

Low-FODMAP Banana Chips

Prep: 10 minutes
Cook: 1 hour
Total time: 1 hour 10 minutes
Serving portions: 4

Nutrition facts:
Calories 61, Total Fat 0.2 g, Saturated Fat 0.1 g, Cholesterol 502 mg, Sodium 1 mg, Total Carbs 15.5 g, Fiber 1.8 g, Sugar 8.3 g, Protein 0.7 g

Ingredients Required

- 2 large-sized bananas, peeled and cut into ¼-inch thick slices

APPETIZER & SNACK RECIPES

Procedure of Cooking

1. Preheat the oven to 250 °F.
2. Line a large-sized baking sheet with baking paper.
3. Place the banana slices onto the baking sheet.
4. Bake them in your oven for about 1 hour. Enjoy!

Low-FODMAP Spicy Pecans

Prep: 10 minutes
Cook: 12 minutes
Total Time: 22 minutes
Serving portions: 16

Nutrition facts:
Calories 125, Total Fat 13 g, Saturated Fat 1.4 g, Cholesterol 0 mg, Sodium 12 mg, Total Carbs 2.4 g, Fiber 1.8 g, Sugar 0.6 g, Protein 1.7 g

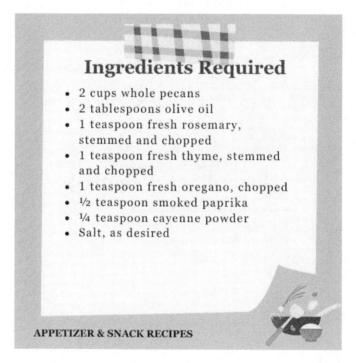

Ingredients Required

- 2 cups whole pecans
- 2 tablespoons olive oil
- 1 teaspoon fresh rosemary, stemmed and chopped
- 1 teaspoon fresh thyme, stemmed and chopped
- 1 teaspoon fresh oregano, chopped
- ½ teaspoon smoked paprika
- ¼ teaspoon cayenne powder
- Salt, as desired

APPETIZER & SNACK RECIPES

Procedure of Cooking

1. Preheat your oven to 350 °F.
2. Arrange a baking paper onto a large-sized baking sheet.
3. In a bowl, place pecans, fresh herbs, spices, and salt. Toss to blend.
4. Put the pecan mixture onto the baking sheet and spread.
5. Roast for about 10-12 minutes, flipping after every 5 minutes.
6. Take out of oven and set the baking sheet aside to cool thoroughly before enjoying them.

Low-FODMAP Berry Gazpacho

Prep: 10 minutes
Total Time: 10 minutes
Serving portions: 6

Nutrition facts:
Calories 77, Total Fat 2.8 g, Saturated Fat 0.2 g, Cholesterol 0 mg, Sodium 121 mg,
Total Carbs 13.3 g, Fiber 4.5 g, Sugar 6.7 g, Protein 1.5 g

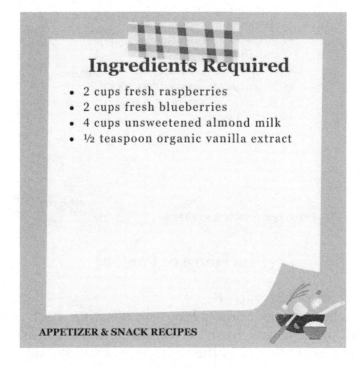

Ingredients Required

- 2 cups fresh raspberries
- 2 cups fresh blueberries
- 4 cups unsweetened almond milk
- ½ teaspoon organic vanilla extract

APPETIZER & SNACK RECIPES

Procedure of Cooking

1. In a clean food processor, put berries, almond milk, and vanilla extract. Process until perfectly smooth.
2. Enjoy immediately.

MAIN DISH RECIPES

Low-FODMAP Salmon & Quinoa Soup

Prep: 15 minutes
Cook: 1 hour 10 minutes
Total Time: 1 hour 25 minutes
Serving portions: 8

Nutrition facts:
Calories 289, Total Fat 14.2 g, Saturated Fat 7.5 g, Cholesterol 31 mg, Sodium 770 mg,
Total Carbs 18.7 g, Fiber 3.5 g, Sugar 2.4 g, Protein 22.9 g

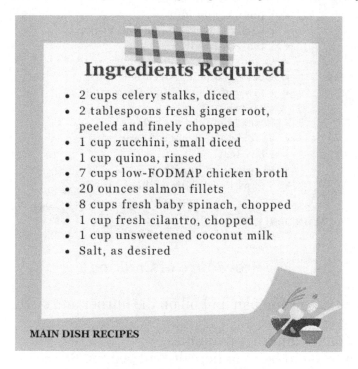

Ingredients Required

- 2 cups celery stalks, diced
- 2 tablespoons fresh ginger root, peeled and finely chopped
- 1 cup zucchini, small diced
- 1 cup quinoa, rinsed
- 7 cups low-FODMAP chicken broth
- 20 ounces salmon fillets
- 8 cups fresh baby spinach, chopped
- 1 cup fresh cilantro, chopped
- 1 cup unsweetened coconut milk
- Salt, as desired

MAIN DISH RECIPES

Procedure of Cooking

1. In a large-sized soup pan, put in celery, ginger root, zucchini, quinoa, and broth. Cook until boiling.
2. Next, adjust the heat to low and cook, covered, for about 45 minutes.
3. Arrange the salmon fillets over the soup mixture.
4. Simmer, covered, for almost 15 minutes.
5. Put in remaining ingredients and cook for 5 minutes.
6. Enjoy hot.

Low-FODMAP Ground Beef & Cabbage Soup

Prep: 15 minutes
Cook: 45 minutes
Total Time: 1 hour
Serving portions: 5

Nutrition facts:
Calories 276, Total Fat 10.2 g, Saturated Fat 3 g, Cholesterol 81 mg, Sodium 711 mg,
Total Carbs 11.1 g, Fiber 3.3 g, Sugar 6 g, Protein 34.3 g

Ingredients Required

- 1 tablespoon olive oil
- 1 large-sized onion, chopped
- 1 pound ground beef
- 2 garlic cloves, peeled and minced
- 1 teaspoon salt
- ½ teaspoon ground pepper
- 4 cups cabbage, shredded
- 1 (15-ounce) can diced tomatoes with juice
- ½ teaspoon dried thyme
- ½ teaspoon dried oregano
- 1 bay leaf
- ½ teaspoon paprika
- 5 cups low-FODMAP beef broth

MAIN DISH RECIPES

Procedure of Cooking

1. In a large-sized soup pan, put oil on the burner and sizzle at medium-high heat.
2. Cook onion for almost 3-5 minutes.
3. Put in the ground beef, garlic, salt, and pepper. Stir to blend.
4. Immediately adjust the heat to medium-high and cook for about 7-8 minutes.
5. Put in the cabbage, tomatoes, herbs, bay leaf, paprika, and broth. Cook until boiling.
6. Next, adjust the heat to low and cook for about 25 minutes.
7. Season with more salt and pepper and enjoy hot.

Low-FODMAP Pork Stew

Prep: 15 minutes
Cook: 1 hour 25 minutes
Total Time: 1 hour 40 minutes
Serving portions: 10

Nutrition facts:
Calories 276, Total Fat 8.3 g, Saturated Fat 1.9 g, Cholesterol 66 mg, Sodium 350 mg, Total Carbs 21.6 g, Fiber 4.2 g, Sugar 5 g, Protein 29 g

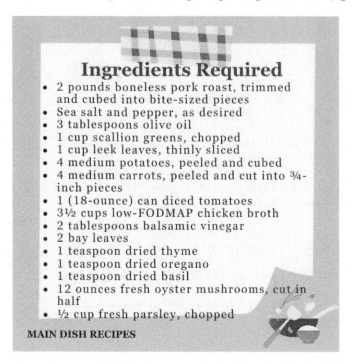

Ingredients Required

- 2 pounds boneless pork roast, trimmed and cubed into bite-sized pieces
- Sea salt and pepper, as desired
- 3 tablespoons olive oil
- 1 cup scallion greens, chopped
- 1 cup leek leaves, thinly sliced
- 4 medium potatoes, peeled and cubed
- 4 medium carrots, peeled and cut into ¾-inch pieces
- 1 (18-ounce) can diced tomatoes
- 3½ cups low-FODMAP chicken broth
- 2 tablespoons balsamic vinegar
- 2 bay leaves
- 1 teaspoon dried thyme
- 1 teaspoon dried oregano
- 1 teaspoon dried basil
- 12 ounces fresh oyster mushrooms, cut in half
- ½ cup fresh parsley, chopped

MAIN DISH RECIPES

Procedure of Cooking

1. In a medium-sized bowl, put in pork cubes, salt, and pepper. Toss to blend.
2. Put oil in a large-sized Dutch oven and sizzle on the burner at medium-high heat.
3. Cook pork cubes in 2 batches for about 2-3 minutes, until browned.
4. Put the browned pork onto a plate.
5. In the same pan, put in scallion greens and leek leaves for about 2-3 minutes.
6. Add potatoes, carrots, tomatoes, broth, vinegar, bay leaves, thyme, oregano, basil, salt, and pepper. Cook until boiling.
7. Next, adjust the heat to low and cook for 5 minutes.
8. Put in the cooked pork and cook, covered, for about 45-50 minutes.
9. Add mushrooms and cook for about 10-15 minutes.
10. Enjoy hot, with the garnishing of parsley.

Low-FODMAP Vegetable Stew

Prep: 15 minutes
Cook: 35 minutes
Total Time: 50 minutes
Serving portions: 4

Nutrition facts:
Calories 330, Total Fat 23.5 g, Saturated Fat 2.6 g, Cholesterol 0 mg, Sodium 1911 mg, Total Carbs 23.6 g, Fiber 7.9 g, Sugar 9.1 g, Protein 11 g

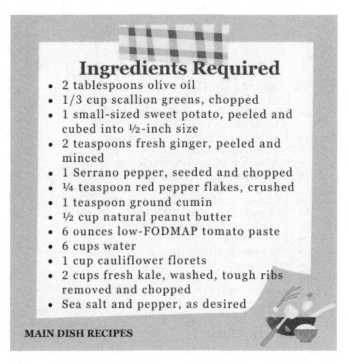

Ingredients Required

- 2 tablespoons olive oil
- 1/3 cup scallion greens, chopped
- 1 small-sized sweet potato, peeled and cubed into ½-inch size
- 2 teaspoons fresh ginger, peeled and minced
- 1 Serrano pepper, seeded and chopped
- ¼ teaspoon red pepper flakes, crushed
- 1 teaspoon ground cumin
- ½ cup natural peanut butter
- 6 ounces low-FODMAP tomato paste
- 6 cups water
- 1 cup cauliflower florets
- 2 cups fresh kale, washed, tough ribs removed and chopped
- Sea salt and pepper, as desired

MAIN DISH RECIPES

Procedure of Cooking

1. In a Dutch oven, put oil on the burner and sizzle at around medium heat.
2. Cook scallion greens for about 2-3 minutes.
3. Add sweet potato and cook for about 5-7 minutes.
4. Add ginger, Serrano pepper, and spices. Cook for 1 minute.
5. Add peanut butter and tomato paste. Cook for 2 minutes.
6. Add water and cook until boiling.
7. Cover and cook for 5 minutes.
8. Put in cauliflower and adjust the heat to low.
9. Simmer for 10 minutes.
10. Put in kale and cook for about 5-8 minutes, until kale is softened.
11. Put in salt and pepper. Enjoy hot.

Low-FODMAP Turkey & Beans Chili

Prep: 15 minutes
Cook: 45 minutes
Total Time: 1 hour
Serving portions: 6

Nutrition facts:
Calories 286, Total Fat 11.2 g, Saturated Fat 2.6 g, Cholesterol 54 mg,
Sodium 292 mg, Total Carbs 27.9 g, Fiber 7.6 g, Sugar 7 g, Protein 21.9 g

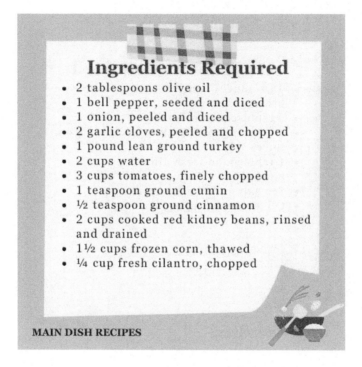

Ingredients Required

- 2 tablespoons olive oil
- 1 bell pepper, seeded and diced
- 1 onion, peeled and diced
- 2 garlic cloves, peeled and chopped
- 1 pound lean ground turkey
- 2 cups water
- 3 cups tomatoes, finely chopped
- 1 teaspoon ground cumin
- ½ teaspoon ground cinnamon
- 2 cups cooked red kidney beans, rinsed and drained
- 1½ cups frozen corn, thawed
- ¼ cup fresh cilantro, chopped

MAIN DISH RECIPES

Procedure of Cooking

1. In a large-sized Dutch oven, heat the olive oil at medium-low heat.
2. Cook bell pepper, onion, and garlic for 5 minutes.
3. Add turkey and cook for about 5-6 minutes, breaking up the chunks with a wooden spoon.
4. Add water, tomatoes, and spices. Cook until boiling on high heat.
5. Adjust the heat to medium-low and add in beans and corn.
6. Simmer, covered, for about 30 minutes, stirring from time to time.
7. Enjoy hot, with the garnishing of cilantro.

Low-FODMAP Lemony Chicken Breasts

Prep: 10 minutes
Cook: 16 minutes
Total Time: 26 minutes
Serving portions: 4

Nutrition facts:
Calories 282, Total Fat 15.5 g, Saturated Fat 3.4 g, Cholesterol 101 mg,
Sodium 138 mg, Total Carbs 1.1 g, Fiber 0.2 g, Sugar 0.2 g, Protein 33 g

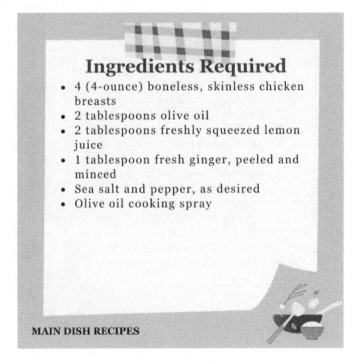

Ingredients Required

- 4 (4-ounce) boneless, skinless chicken breasts
- 2 tablespoons olive oil
- 2 tablespoons freshly squeezed lemon juice
- 1 tablespoon fresh ginger, peeled and minced
- Sea salt and pepper, as desired
- Olive oil cooking spray

MAIN DISH RECIPES

Procedure of Cooking

1. In a large-sized bowl, put in oil, lemon juice, ginger, salt, and pepper. Whisk until blended thoroughly.
2. In a large-sized resealable plastic bag, place the chicken and marinade.
3. Seal the bag and shake to coat well.
4. Put the bag in your refrigerator to marinate overnight.
5. Preheat the grill to medium heat.
6. Grease the grill grate with cooking spray.
7. Take out the chicken from the bag and discard the marinade.
8. Place the chicken onto the grill grate and grill, covered, for about 5-8 minutes on each side.
9. Enjoy hot.

Low-FODMAP Chicken Roulade

Prep: 15 minutes
Cook: 17 minutes
Total time: 32 minutes
Serving portions: 4

Nutrition facts:
Calories 385, Total Fat 22.8 g, Saturated Fat 8.1 g, Cholesterol 124 mg,
Sodium 416 mg, Total Carbs 2.7 g, Fiber 1 g, Sugar 1.3 g, Protein 42.3 g

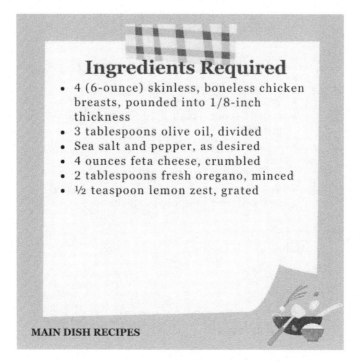

Ingredients Required

- 4 (6-ounce) skinless, boneless chicken breasts, pounded into 1/8-inch thickness
- 3 tablespoons olive oil, divided
- Sea salt and pepper, as desired
- 4 ounces feta cheese, crumbled
- 2 tablespoons fresh oregano, minced
- ½ teaspoon lemon zest, grated

MAIN DISH RECIPES

Procedure of Cooking

1. Preheat your oven to 450 °F.
2. Brush the chicken breasts with 1 tablespoon of oil and then season with salt and pepper.
3. Arrange the chicken breasts onto a smooth surface.
4. Top each chicken breast with feta, followed by oregano and lemon zest, leaving edges clear.
5. Roll each breast like a jellyroll to seal the filling securely.
6. With kitchen twine, tie each roll at 1-inch intervals.
7. Heat remaining oil and add chicken breasts to cook for about 10 minutes.
8. Take off the flat-bottomed wok of chicken rolls from burner.
9. Arrange the rolls into a baking dish.
10. Bake in your oven for about 5-7 minutes.
11. Enjoy hot.

Low-FODMAP Ground Turkey with Green Beans

Prep: 10 minutes
Cook: 22 minutes
Total Time: 32 minutes
Serving portions: 6

Nutrition facts:
Calories 224, Total Fat 13 g, Saturated Fat 3.3 g, Cholesterol 81 mg, Sodium 149 mg, Total Carbs 4.7 g, Fiber 2 g, Sugar 0.8 g, Protein 23.6 g

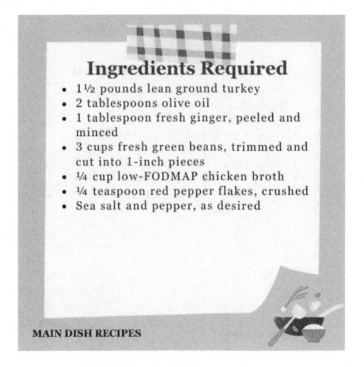

Ingredients Required

- 1½ pounds lean ground turkey
- 2 tablespoons olive oil
- 1 tablespoon fresh ginger, peeled and minced
- 3 cups fresh green beans, trimmed and cut into 1-inch pieces
- ¼ cup low-FODMAP chicken broth
- ¼ teaspoon red pepper flakes, crushed
- Sea salt and pepper, as desired

MAIN DISH RECIPES

Procedure of Cooking

1. Put an anti-sticking, flat-bottomed wok on the burner and sizzle at medium-high heat.
2. Cook turkey for about 6-8 minutes.
3. Put in the ginger and cook for 1 minute.
4. Put in green beans and stir to blend.
5. Put in the broth, red pepper flakes, salt, and pepper. Cook until boiling.
6. Next, adjust the heat to medium-low and cook for about 6-8 minutes, stirring regularly.
7. Enjoy hot.

Low-FODMAP Herbed Flank Steak

Prep: 10 minutes
Cook: 20 minutes
Total: 30 minutes
Serving portions: 6

Nutrition facts:
Calories 221, Total Fat 9.5 g, Saturated Fat 3.9 g, Cholesterol 62 mg, Sodium 91 mg,
Total Carbs 0.1 g, Fiber 0.1 g, Sugar 0 g, Protein 31.6 g

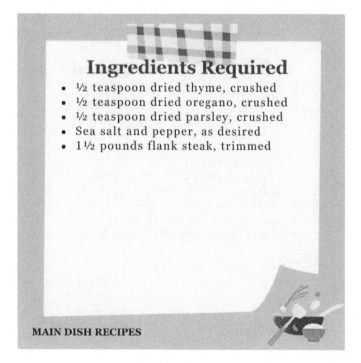

Ingredients Required

- ½ teaspoon dried thyme, crushed
- ½ teaspoon dried oregano, crushed
- ½ teaspoon dried parsley, crushed
- Sea salt and pepper, as desired
- 1½ pounds flank steak, trimmed

MAIN DISH RECIPES

Procedure of Cooking

1. In a large-sized bowl, put in the dried herbs, salt, and pepper. Blend thoroughly.
2. Put in the steaks and rub with herb mixture generously.
3. Set it aside for about 15-20 minutes.
4. Preheat the grill to medium heat.
5. Grease the grill grate.
6. Place the steak onto the grill over medium coals and cook for about 18-20 minutes, flipping once halfway through.
7. Take the steak from grill and place onto a cutting board to rest for 10 minutes before slicing.

Low-FODMAP Beef with Bell Peppers

Prep: 15 minutes
Cook: 20 minutes
Total Time: 35 minutes
Serving portions: 6

Nutrition facts:
Calories 230, Total Fat 12 g, Saturated Fat 2.8 g, Cholesterol 68 mg, Sodium 111 mg, Total Carbs 6.5 g, Fiber 1.3 g, Sugar 3.8 g, Protein 24 g

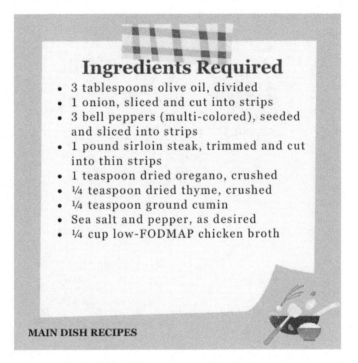

Ingredients Required

- 3 tablespoons olive oil, divided
- 1 onion, sliced and cut into strips
- 3 bell peppers (multi-colored), seeded and sliced into strips
- 1 pound sirloin steak, trimmed and cut into thin strips
- 1 teaspoon dried oregano, crushed
- ¼ teaspoon dried thyme, crushed
- ¼ teaspoon ground cumin
- Sea salt and pepper, as desired
- ¼ cup low-FODMAP chicken broth

MAIN DISH RECIPES

Procedure of Cooking

1. Heat 1 tablespoon of oil in a flat-bottomed wok at medium-high heat.
2. Cook onion and bell pepper slices for about 4-5 minutes, or until softened.
3. With a slotted spoon, put the peppers mixture onto a plate.
4. Melt the remaining butter in the same flat-bottomed wok at medium-high heat.
5. Cook beef for about 4-5 minutes, stirring regularly.
6. Put in the thyme, spices, salt, pepper, and broth. Cook until boiling.
7. Add in the pepper mixture and stir to blend.
8. Next, adjust the heat to medium and cook for about 3-5 minutes, stirring from time to time.
9. Enjoy immediately.

Low-FODMAP Parsley Pork Tenderloin

Prep: 10 minutes
Cook: 22 minutes
Total Time: 32 minutes
Serving portions: 4

Nutrition facts:
Calories 194, Total Fat 7.6 g, Saturated Fat 1.9 g, Cholesterol 83 mg, Sodium 119 mg, Total Carbs 0.2 g, Fiber 0.1 g, Sugar 0.1 g, Protein 29.8 g

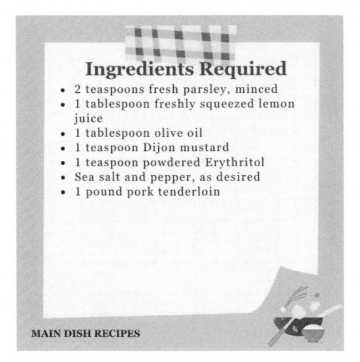

Ingredients Required

- 2 teaspoons fresh parsley, minced
- 1 tablespoon freshly squeezed lemon juice
- 1 tablespoon olive oil
- 1 teaspoon Dijon mustard
- 1 teaspoon powdered Erythritol
- Sea salt and pepper, as desired
- 1 pound pork tenderloin

MAIN DISH RECIPES

Procedure of Cooking

1. Preheat your oven to 400 °F.
2. Grease a large-sized rimmed baking sheet.
3. In a mixing bowl, place parsley and remaining ingredients, except the pork tenderloin and whisk until blended thoroughly.
4. Add pork tenderloin and coat with the mixture generously.
5. Arrange the pork tenderloin onto the greased baking sheet.
6. Bake it in your oven for about 20-22 minutes.
7. Take the baking sheet out of the oven and place the pork tenderloin onto a cutting board to rest for 5 minutes.
8. Cut the pork tenderloin into ¾-inch-thick slices and enjoy.

Low-FODMAP Chickpeas & Spinach Curry

Prep: 15 minutes
Cook: 55 minutes
Total Time: 1 hour 10 minutes
Serving portions: 8

Nutrition facts:
Calories 141, Total Fat 5.3 g, Saturated Fat 0.8 g, Cholesterol 0 mg, Sodium 252 mg, Total Carbs 18.7 g, Fiber 5.5 g, Sugar 5.7 g, Protein 6.4 g

Ingredients Required

- 2 tablespoons olive oil
- 1 cup scallion greens, chopped
- 2 cups carrots, peeled and chopped
- 1 teaspoon ground cumin
- 1 teaspoon ground coriander
- 1 teaspoon red pepper flakes
- 3 large tomatoes, peeled, seeded, and finely chopped
- 2 cups low-FODMAP vegetable broth
- ¾ cup cooked chickpeas
- 4 cups fresh spinach, washed thoroughly and chopped
- 1 tablespoon freshly squeezed lemon juice
- Sea salt and pepper, as desired

MAIN DISH RECIPES

Procedure of Cooking

1. In a saucepan, put oil on the burner and sizzle at medium heat.
2. Cook carrots and celery for 5 minutes.
3. Put in the spices and cook for 1 minute.
4. Add lentils, tomatoes, and water. Cook until boiling.
5. Next adjust the heat to low and cook, covered, for about 40 minutes.
6. Put in spinach, salt, and pepper. Cook for almost 3-5 minutes.
7. Enjoy hot.

Low-FODMAP Dill Salmon

Prep: 10 minutes
Cook: 25 minutes
Total Time: 35 minutes
Serving portions: 3

Nutrition facts:
Calories 307, Total Fat 15.7 g, Saturated Fat 3.7 g, Cholesterol 99 mg, Sodium 121 mg, Total Carbs 2.9 g, Fiber 0.9 g, Sugar 0.2 g, Protein 38.9 g

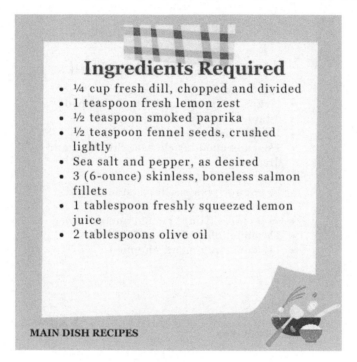

Ingredients Required

- ¼ cup fresh dill, chopped and divided
- 1 teaspoon fresh lemon zest
- ½ teaspoon smoked paprika
- ½ teaspoon fennel seeds, crushed lightly
- Sea salt and pepper, as desired
- 3 (6-ounce) skinless, boneless salmon fillets
- 1 tablespoon freshly squeezed lemon juice
- 2 tablespoons olive oil

MAIN DISH RECIPES

Procedure of Cooking

1. In a bowl, place 2 tablespoons of dill, lemon zest, paprika, fennel seeds, salt, and pepper. Blend thoroughly.
2. Season the salmon fillets with dill mixture evenly and then drizzle with lemon juice.
3. In a large-sized, flat-bottomed wok, put oil on the burner and sizzle at medium heat.
4. In the flat-bottomed wok, place the salmon fillets.
5. Next, adjust the heat to low and cook for almost 20 minutes.
6. Flip the salmon fillets and cook for 5 minutes more.
7. With a slotted spoon, put the salmon fillets onto a paper towel-lined plate to drain.
8. Serve immediately, with the garnishing of remaining fresh dill.

Low-FODMAP Seafood Casserole

Prep: 15 minutes
Cook: 1 hour 5 minutes
Total Time: 1 hour 20 minutes
Serving portions: 8

Nutrition facts:
Calories 267, Total Fat 17.9 g, Saturated Fat 10.9 g, Cholesterol 166 mg,
Sodium 487 mg, Total Carbs 2.6 g, Fiber 0.4 g, Sugar 0.5 g, Protein 22.9 g

Ingredients Required

- 2½ cup water
- 2 cups celery, trimmed and chopped
- 3 tablespoons unsalted butter
- 1 cup heavy cream
- 1½ cups cheddar cheese, shredded and divided.
- Sea salt and pepper, as desired
- ½ pound fresh scallops, side muscles removed
- ½ pound shrimp, peeled and deveined
- 1½ cups lobster meat, chopped
- 1½ cups crab meat, chopped

MAIN DISH RECIPES

Procedure of Cooking

1. Preheat your oven to 325 °F.
2. In a large-sized saucepan, place the water at medium-highand heat until boiling.
3. Put in the celery and cook for almost 6 minutes.
4. With a slotted spoon, place the cooked celery into a large-sized bowl.
5. In the same pan of boiling water, add in the scallops at low heat and cook for 3 minutes.
6. With a slotted spoon, put the scallops into the bowl of celery.
7. Again, in the same saucepan of boiling water, add the shrimp at low heat and cook for 4 minutes.
8. With a slotted spoon, add the shrimp into the bowl of celery.
9. Reserve ¾ cup of the cooking water and set it aside.
10. Into the bowl of shrimp mixture, put in the lobster and crab meat. Blend thoroughly.
11. In a large-sized, flat-bottomed wok, place the butter on the burner at medium heat and cook until it starts to brown.
12. Slowly add the cream and reserved cooking water, stirring regularly until blended thoroughly.
13. Cook for about 1-2 minutes.
14. Into the sauce, add 1 cup of cheese and stir until melted completely.
15. Add in the seafood mixture, salt, and pepper. Take off the burner.
16. Place the mixture into a 9x13-inch baking dish evenly and top with the remaining cheddar cheese.
17. Bake it in your oven for about 35-45 minutes, until bubbly and browned.
18. Take the baking dish from oven and let it cool for almost 5 minutes before enjoying it.

Low-FODMAP Lentil & Pumpkin Curry

Prep: 15 minutes
Cook: 1½ hours
Total Time: 1¾ hours
Serving portions: 8

Nutrition facts:
Calories 263, Total Fat 3 g, Saturated Fat 0.5 g, Cholesterol 0 mg, Sodium 53 mg,
Total Carbs 47 g, Fiber 20 g, Sugar 9.7 g, Protein 14.7 g

Ingredients Required

- 8 cups water
- ½ teaspoon ground turmeric
- 1 cup brown lentils
- 1 cup red lentils
- 1 tablespoon olive oil
- 1 large-sized white onion, peeled and chopped
- 3 garlic cloves, peeled and minced
- 2 tomatoes, seeded and chopped
- 1½ tablespoons curry powder
- ¼ teaspoon ground cloves
- 2 teaspoons ground cumin
- 3 carrots, peeled and chopped
- 3 cups pumpkin, peeled, seeded, and cubed into 1-inch sized pieces
- 1 granny smith apple, cored and chopped
- 2 cups fresh spinach, chopped
- Sea salt and pepper, as desired

MAIN DISH RECIPES

Procedure of Cooking

1. In a large-sized saucepan, put in the water, turmeric, and lentils at high heat and cook until boiling.
2. Next, adjust the heat to medium-low and cook, covered, for 30 minutes.
3. Drain the lentils, reserving 2½ cups of the cooking liquid.
4. Meanwhile, in another large pan, put in oil and sizzle on medium heat.
5. Cook onion for about 2-3 minutes.
6. Add the garlic and cook for 1 minute.
7. Put in the tomatoes and cook for 5 minutes.
8. Add in the curry powder and spices. Cook for 1 minute.
9. Put in the carrots, potatoes, pumpkin, cooked lentils, and reserved cooking liquid. Cook until boiling.
10. Next, adjust the heat to medium-low and cook, covered, for about 40-45 minutes.
11. Add in the apple and spinach. Cook for 15 minutes, until spinach is softened.
12. Add in the salt and pepper. Remove from burner.
13. Enjoy hot.

VEGETABLES & SALADS RECIPES

Vegetable Lettuce Wraps

Prep: 15 minutes
Total Time: 15 minutes
Serving portions: 3

Nutrition facts:
Calories 30, Total Fat 0.2 g, Saturated Fat 0 g, Cholesterol 0 mg, Sodium 77 mg, Total Carbs 7.1 g, Fiber 1.6 g, Sugar 4 g, Protein 0.9 g

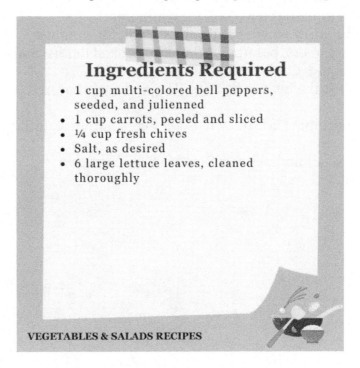

Ingredients Required
- 1 cup multi-colored bell peppers, seeded, and julienned
- 1 cup carrots, peeled and sliced
- ¼ cup fresh chives
- Salt, as desired
- 6 large lettuce leaves, cleaned thoroughly

VEGETABLES & SALADS RECIPES

Procedure of Cooking

1. In a large-sized bowl, put in the bell peppers, carrots, chives, and salt. Blend thoroughly.
2. Arrange the lettuce leaves onto serving plates.
3. Divide the peppers and carrot mixture onto each lettuce leaf evenly.
4. Enjoy immediately.

Stuffed Zucchini

Prep: 15 minutes
Cook: 18 minutes
Total Time: 23 minutes
Serving portions: 8

Nutrition facts:
Calories 59, Total Fat 3.2 g, Saturated Fat 1.6 g, Cholesterol 8 mg, Sodium 208 mg, Total Carbs 6.1 g, Fiber 1.9 g, Sugar 3.2 g, Protein 2.9 g

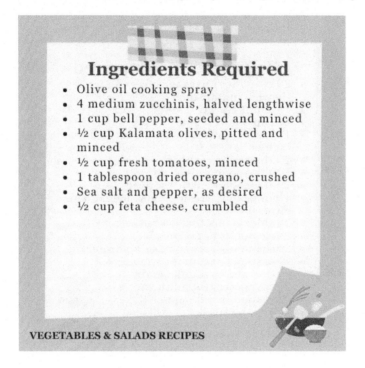

Ingredients Required

- Olive oil cooking spray
- 4 medium zucchinis, halved lengthwise
- 1 cup bell pepper, seeded and minced
- ½ cup Kalamata olives, pitted and minced
- ½ cup fresh tomatoes, minced
- 1 tablespoon dried oregano, crushed
- Sea salt and pepper, as desired
- ½ cup feta cheese, crumbled

VEGETABLES & SALADS RECIPES

Procedure of Cooking

1. Preheat your oven to 350 °F.
2. Grease a large-sized baking sheet with cooking spray.
3. With a melon baller, scoop out the flesh of each zucchini half. Discard the flesh.
4. In a bowl, blend together the bell pepper, olives, tomatoes, oregano, salt and pepper.
5. Stuff each zucchini half with the vegetable mixture evenly.
6. Arrange zucchini halves onto the baking sheet and bake them in your oven for 15 minutes.
7. Next, set the oven to broil on high.
8. Top each zucchini half with feta cheese and broil for 3 minutes, until browned on top.
9. Enjoy hot.

Spinach with Cottage Cheese

Prep: 15 minutes
Cook: 25 minutes
Total Time: 40 minutes
Serving portions: 8

Nutrition facts:
Calories 121, Net Carbs 5.2 g, Total Fat 6.1 g, Saturated Fat 3.6 g, Cholesterol 15 mg, Sodium 334 mg, Total Carbs 7.4 g, Fiber 2.2 g, Sugar 0.9 g, Protein 10.5 g

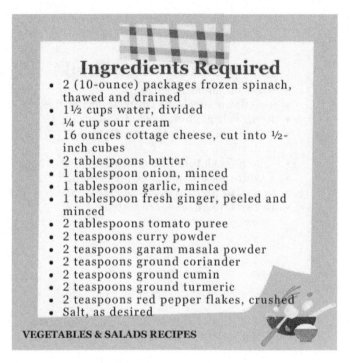

Ingredients Required

- 2 (10-ounce) packages frozen spinach, thawed and drained
- 1½ cups water, divided
- ¼ cup sour cream
- 16 ounces cottage cheese, cut into ½-inch cubes
- 2 tablespoons butter
- 1 tablespoon onion, minced
- 1 tablespoon garlic, minced
- 1 tablespoon fresh ginger, peeled and minced
- 2 tablespoons tomato puree
- 2 teaspoons curry powder
- 2 teaspoons garam masala powder
- 2 teaspoons ground coriander
- 2 teaspoons ground cumin
- 2 teaspoons ground turmeric
- 2 teaspoons red pepper flakes, crushed
- Salt, as desired

VEGETABLES & SALADS RECIPES

Procedure of Cooking

1. Place spinach, ½ cup of water, and sour cream into a clean blender and process until pureed.
2. Put the spinach puree into a bowl and set it aside.
3. In a large-sized anti-sticking, flat-bottomed wok, put in butter and let it melt on the burner at medium-low heat.
4. Cook the onion, garlic, ginger, tomato puree, spices, and salt for about 2-3 minutes.
5. Add in the spinach puree and remaining water. Stir to blend.
6. Adjust the heat to medium and cook for about 3-5 minutes.
7. Add cheese cubes and stir to blend.
8. Adjust the heat to low and cook for about 10-15 minutes.
9. Enjoy hot.

Banana Curry

Prep: 15 minutes
Cook: 15 minutes
Total Time: 30 minutes
Serving portions: 4

Nutrition facts:
Calories 216, Total Fat 9.1 g, Saturated Fat 1.7 g, Cholesterol 2 mg, Sodium 105 mg,
Total Carbs 32 g, Fiber 6.5 g, Sugar 16.4 g, Protein 6.2 g

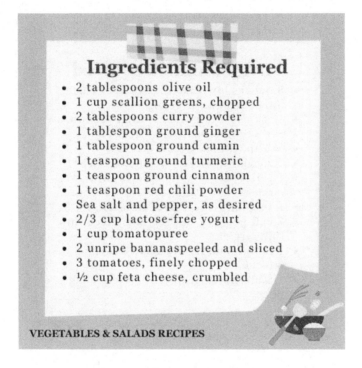

Ingredients Required
- 2 tablespoons olive oil
- 1 cup scallion greens, chopped
- 2 tablespoons curry powder
- 1 tablespoon ground ginger
- 1 tablespoon ground cumin
- 1 teaspoon ground turmeric
- 1 teaspoon ground cinnamon
- 1 teaspoon red chili powder
- Sea salt and pepper, as desired
- 2/3 cup lactose-free yogurt
- 1 cup tomatopuree
- 2 unripe bananaspeeled and sliced
- 3 tomatoes, finely chopped
- ½ cup feta cheese, crumbled

VEGETABLES & SALADS RECIPES

Procedure of Cooking

1. In a large-sized saucepan, put oil on the burner and sizzle at medium heat.
2. Cook scallion greens for about 3-4 minutes.
3. Put in the curry powder and spices. Cook for almost 1 minute.
4. Add in the yogurt and tomato sauce. Cook until boiling.
5. Put in the bananas and cook for 3 minutes.
6. Add in the tomatoes and cook for about 1-2 minutes.
7. Enjoy hot.

Mixed Vegetable Combo

Prep: 15 minutes
Cook: 45 minutes
Total Time: 1 hour
Serving portions: 4

Nutrition facts:
Calories 207, Total Fat 11.4 g, Saturated Fat 1.7 g, Cholesterol 0 mg, Sodium 111 mg,
Total Carbs 26.7 g, Fiber 8.8 g, Sugar 15.4 g, Protein 5.7 g

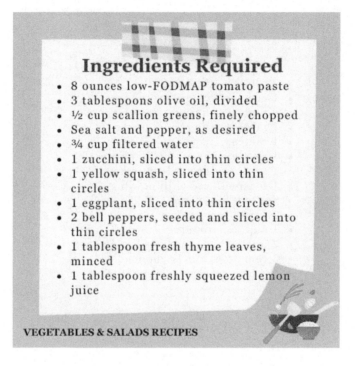

Ingredients Required
- 8 ounces low-FODMAP tomato paste
- 3 tablespoons olive oil, divided
- ½ cup scallion greens, finely chopped
- Sea salt and pepper, as desired
- ¾ cup filtered water
- 1 zucchini, sliced into thin circles
- 1 yellow squash, sliced into thin circles
- 1 eggplant, sliced into thin circles
- 2 bell peppers, seeded and sliced into thin circles
- 1 tablespoon fresh thyme leaves, minced
- 1 tablespoon freshly squeezed lemon juice

VEGETABLES & SALADS RECIPES

Procedure of Cooking

1. Preheat your oven to 375 °F.
2. In a small-sized bowl, put in the tomato paste, 1 tablespoon of oil, scallion greens, salt, and pepper. Blend.
3. In the bottom of a 10x10-inch baking dish, spread the tomato paste mixture evenly.
4. Arrange alternating vegetable slices, starting at the outer edge of the baking dish and working concentrically towards the center.
5. Drizzle the vegetables with the remaining oil. Sprinkle with salt and pepper, followed by the thyme.
6. Arrange a piece of parchment paper over the vegetables.
7. Bake it in your oven for about 45 minutes.
8. Enjoy hot.

Egg Salad

Prep: 10 minutes
Total Time: 10 minutes
Serving portions: 2

Nutrition facts:
Calories 216, Total Fat 14.2 g, Saturated Fat 3.8 g, Cholesterol 333 mg, Sodium 332 mg, Total Carbs 8.9 g, Fiber 0.7 g, Sugar 4.6 g, Protein 13.4 g

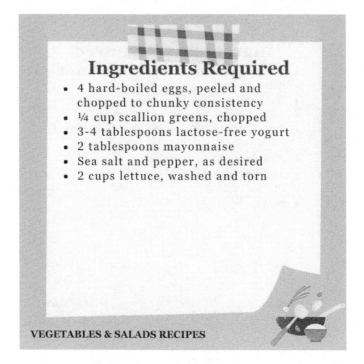

Ingredients Required

- 4 hard-boiled eggs, peeled and chopped to chunky consistency
- ¼ cup scallion greens, chopped
- 3-4 tablespoons lactose-free yogurt
- 2 tablespoons mayonnaise
- Sea salt and pepper, as desired
- 2 cups lettuce, washed and torn

VEGETABLES & SALADS RECIPES

Procedure of Cooking

1. In a medium-sized salad bowl, put in egg pieces, scallion greens, yogurt, mayonnaise, salt, and pepper. Gently stir to blend.
2. Line a serving plate with lettuce evenly
3. Top with egg mixture and enjoy immediately.

Cucumber & Tomato Salad

Prep: 15 minutes
Total Time: 15 minutes
Serving portions: 4

Nutrition facts:
Calories 92, Total Fat 7.4 g, Saturated Fat 1.1 g, Cholesterol 0 mg, Sodium 58 mg, Total Carbs 6.8 g, Fiber 1.8 g, Sugar 3.6 g, Protein 1.7 g

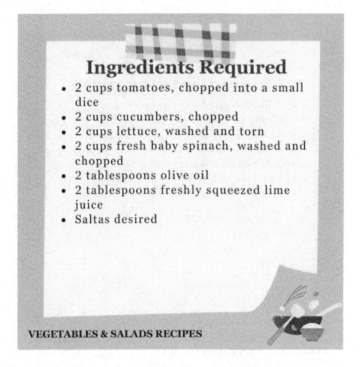

Ingredients Required

- 2 cups tomatoes, chopped into a small dice
- 2 cups cucumbers, chopped
- 2 cups lettuce, washed and torn
- 2 cups fresh baby spinach, washed and chopped
- 2 tablespoons olive oil
- 2 tablespoons freshly squeezed lime juice
- Saltas desired

VEGETABLES & SALADS RECIPES

Procedure of Cooking

1. Place all ingredients in a large-sized serving bowl and gently toss to combine.
2. Enjoy immediately.

Berry Salad

Prep: 15 minutes
All the time: 15 minutes
Serving portions: 4

Nutrition facts:
Calories 177, Total Fat 16.1 g, Saturated Fat 2 g, Cholesterol 0 mg, Sodium 43 mg, Total Carbs 8.9 g, Fiber 1.9 g, Sugar 5.6 g, Protein 1.3 g

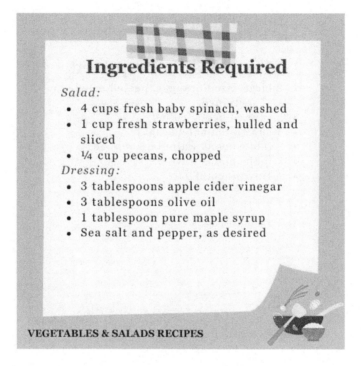

Ingredients Required

Salad:
- 4 cups fresh baby spinach, washed
- 1 cup fresh strawberries, hulled and sliced
- ¼ cup pecans, chopped

Dressing:
- 3 tablespoons apple cider vinegar
- 3 tablespoons olive oil
- 1 tablespoon pure maple syrup
- Sea salt and pepper, as desired

VEGETABLES & SALADS RECIPES

Procedure of Cooking

1. For the salad: place spinach, strawberries, and pecans in a large-sized bowl and blend thoroughly.
2. For the dressing: place vinegar, olive oil, maple syrup, salt, and pepper in a small-sized bowl and whisk until blended thoroughly.
3. Pour the dressing over the salad and toss it all to coat well.
4. Enjoy immediately.

Orange & Beet Salad

Prep: 15 minutes
Total Time: 15 minutes
Serving portions: 4

Nutrition facts:
Calories 184, Total Fat 13.1 g, Saturated Fat 1.7 g, Cholesterol 0 mg, Sodium 83 mg, Total Carbs 16.9 g, Fiber 3.8 g, Sugar 13 g, Protein 3.2 g

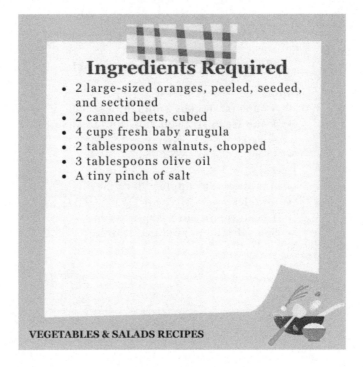

Ingredients Required

- 2 large-sized oranges, peeled, seeded, and sectioned
- 2 canned beets, cubed
- 4 cups fresh baby arugula
- 2 tablespoons walnuts, chopped
- 3 tablespoons olive oil
- A tiny pinch of salt

VEGETABLES & SALADS RECIPES

Procedure of Cooking

1. In a salad bowl, place all ingredients and gently toss to coat.
2. Enjoy immediately.

Avocado Salad

Prep: 15 minutes
Total Time: 15 minutes
Serving portions: 4

Nutrition facts:
Calories 268, Total Fat 23.5 g, Saturated Fat 4.7 g, Cholesterol 0 mg, Sodium 84 mg,
Total Carbs 15.4 g, Fiber 8.7 g, Sugar 4.1 g, Protein 3.8 g

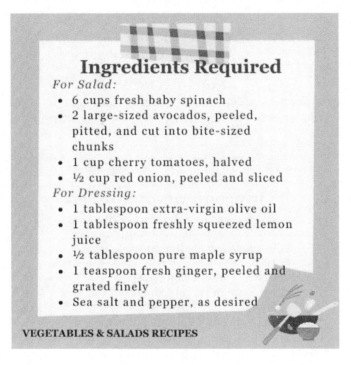

Ingredients Required

For Salad:
- 6 cups fresh baby spinach
- 2 large-sized avocados, peeled, pitted, and cut into bite-sized chunks
- 1 cup cherry tomatoes, halved
- ½ cup red onion, peeled and sliced

For Dressing:
- 1 tablespoon extra-virgin olive oil
- 1 tablespoon freshly squeezed lemon juice
- ½ tablespoon pure maple syrup
- 1 teaspoon fresh ginger, peeled and grated finely
- Sea salt and pepper, as desired

VEGETABLES & SALADS RECIPES

Procedure of Cooking

1. For the salad: place spinach, avocados, tomatoes, and onion in a large-sized bowl. Blend thoroughly.
2. For the dressing: place oil and remaining ingredients in a small-sized bowl and whisk until blended thoroughly.
3. Pour the dressing over the salad and toss it all to coat well.
4. Enjoy immediately.

SIDE DISHES RECIPES

Low-FODMAP Parsley Mushrooms

Prep: 10 minutes
Cook: 15 minutes
Total Time: 25 minutes
Serving portions: 2

Nutrition facts:
Calories 163, Total Fat 14.5 g, Saturated Fat 2 g, Cholesterol 0 mg, Sodium 89 mg, Total Carbs 6.9 g, Fiber 2 g, Sugar 3.4 g, Protein 5.6 g

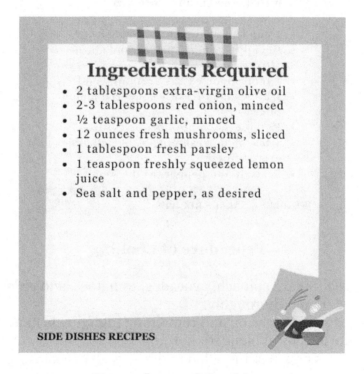

Ingredients Required

- 2 tablespoons extra-virgin olive oil
- 2-3 tablespoons red onion, minced
- ½ teaspoon garlic, minced
- 12 ounces fresh mushrooms, sliced
- 1 tablespoon fresh parsley
- 1 teaspoon freshly squeezed lemon juice
- Sea salt and pepper, as desired

SIDE DISHES RECIPES

Procedure of Cooking

1. In a flat-bottomed wok, put oil on the burner and sizzle at medium heat.
2. Cook onion and garlic for 3-4 minutes.
3. Put in the mushrooms and cook for 8-10 minutes.
4. Put in the parsley, lemon juice, salt, and pepper. Remove from burner.
5. Enjoy hot.

Low-FODMAP Stir Fry Broccoli

Prep: 10 minutes
Cook: 9 minutes
Total Time: 19 minutes
Serving portions: 3

Nutrition facts:
Calories 100, Total Fat 7.9 g, Saturated Fat 0.9 g, Cholesterol 0 mg, Sodium 608 mg, Total Carbs 6.4 g, Fiber 2.5 g, Sugar 2.1 g, Protein 3.7 g

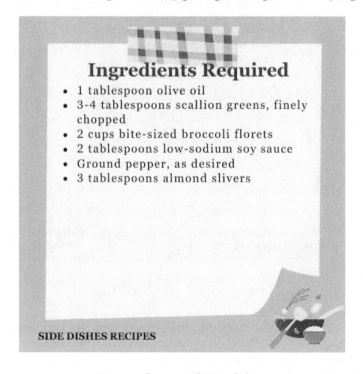

Ingredients Required

- 1 tablespoon olive oil
- 3-4 tablespoons scallion greens, finely chopped
- 2 cups bite-sized broccoli florets
- 2 tablespoons low-sodium soy sauce
- Ground pepper, as desired
- 3 tablespoons almond slivers

SIDE DISHES RECIPES

Procedure of Cooking

1. In a large-sized, flat-bottomed wok, put oil on the burner and sizzle at medium heat.
2. Cook the scallion greens for about 1-2 minutes.
3. Put in the broccoli and stir fry for 2 minutes.
4. Put in the soy sauce and pepper. Stir fry for about 4-5 minutes.
5. Add almonds and enjoy hot.

Low-FODMAP Lemony Kale

Prep: 10 minutes
Cook: 15 minutes
Total Time: 25 minutes
Serving portions: 6

Nutrition facts:
Calories 108, Total Fat 2.4 g, Saturated Fat 0.3 g, Cholesterol 0 mg, Sodium 96 mg, Total Carbs 19.3 g, Fiber 2.7 g, Sugar 2.4 g, Protein 4.8 g

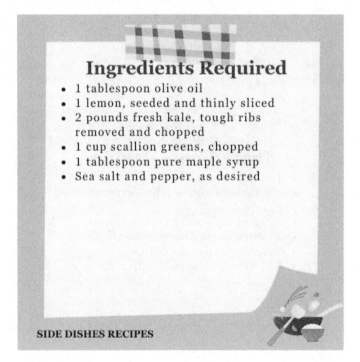

Ingredients Required

- 1 tablespoon olive oil
- 1 lemon, seeded and thinly sliced
- 2 pounds fresh kale, tough ribs removed and chopped
- 1 cup scallion greens, chopped
- 1 tablespoon pure maple syrup
- Sea salt and pepper, as desired

SIDE DISHES RECIPES

Procedure of Cooking

1. In a large-sized, flat-bottomed wok, put oil on the burner and sizzle at medium heat.
2. Cook the lemon slices for 5 minutes.
3. With a slotted spoon, take out the lemon slices.
4. In the same cooking wok, put in the kale, scallion greens, maple syrup, salt, and pepper. Cook for about 8-10 minutes, stirring from time to time.
5. Enjoy hot.

Low-FODMAP Kale with Pine Nuts & Cranberries

Prep: 10 minutes
Cook: 14 minutes
Total Time: 24 minutes
Serving portions: 6

Nutrition facts:
Calories 196, Total Fat 12.2 g, Saturated Fat 1.4 g, Cholesterol 0 mg, Sodium 93 mg,
Total Carbs 19.3 g, Fiber 2.9 g, Sugar 1.3 g, Protein 5.6 g

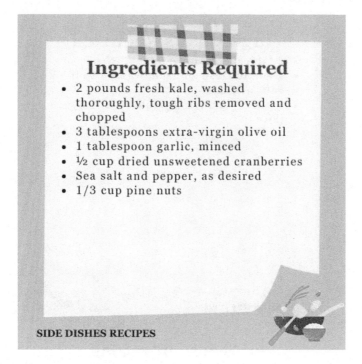

Ingredients Required

- 2 pounds fresh kale, washed thoroughly, tough ribs removed and chopped
- 3 tablespoons extra-virgin olive oil
- 1 tablespoon garlic, minced
- ½ cup dried unsweetened cranberries
- Sea salt and pepper, as desired
- 1/3 cup pine nuts

SIDE DISHES RECIPES

Procedure of Cooking

1. In a large-sized pan of boiling salted water, cook the kale for about 5-7 minutes.
2. In a colander, drain the kale and immediately put into an ice bath.
3. Drain the kale and set it aside.
4. In a flat-bottomed wok, put oil on the burner and sizzle on medium heat.
5. Cook the garlic for almost 1 minute.
6. Add kale, cranberries, salt, and pepper. Cook for about 4-6 minutes, tossing regularly with tongs.
7. Put in the pine nuts and enjoy hot.

Low-FODMAP Lemony Spinach

Prep: 10 minutes
Cook: 5 minutes
Total Time: 15 minutes
Serving portions: 3

Nutrition facts:
Calories 116, Total Fat 10 g, Saturated Fat 1.5 g, Cholesterol 0 mg, Sodium 171 mg, Total Carbs 5.6 g, Fiber 3.4 g, Sugar 0.8 g, Protein 4.4 g

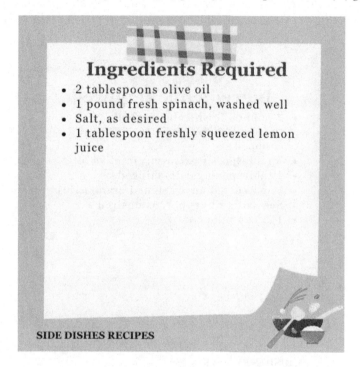

Ingredients Required

- 2 tablespoons olive oil
- 1 pound fresh spinach, washed well
- Salt, as desired
- 1 tablespoon freshly squeezed lemon juice

SIDE DISHES RECIPES

Procedure of Cooking

1. Put oil in an anti-sticking, flat-bottomed wok on burner and sizzle at about medium-high heat.
2. Blend in the spinach and immediately cover the cooking pan.
3. Cook for 2 minutes, flipping the spinach once halfway through.
4. Uncover and drain the spinach completely.
5. Put in the salt and cook for almost 1 minute, stirring regularly.
6. Put in lemon juice and enjoy hot.

Low-FODMAP Garlicky Bok Choy

Prep: 15 minutes
Cook: 10 minutes
Total Time: 25 minutes
Serving portions: 4

Nutrition facts:
Calories 73, Total Fat 5.1 g, Saturated Fat 0.8 g, Cholesterol 0 mg, Sodium 586 mg,
Total Carbs 5.5 g, Fiber 1.9 g, Sugar 2.2 g, Protein 3.4 g

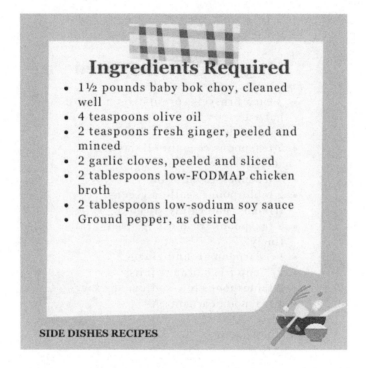

Ingredients Required

- 1½ pounds baby bok choy, cleaned well
- 4 teaspoons olive oil
- 2 teaspoons fresh ginger, peeled and minced
- 2 garlic cloves, peeled and sliced
- 2 tablespoons low-FODMAP chicken broth
- 2 tablespoons low-sodium soy sauce
- Ground pepper, as desired

SIDE DISHES RECIPES

Procedure of Cooking

1. Trim bases of bok choy and separate outer leaves from stalks, leaving the smallest inner leaves attached.
2. In a large-sized cast-iron, flat-bottomed wok, put oil on the burner and sizzle at medium-high heat.
3. Cook the ginger and garlic for 1 minute.
4. Put in the bok choy leaves and stalks. Cook for 1 minute, tossing with tongs.
5. Put in the broth, soy sauce, and pepper. Cook for about 2-3 minutes, tossing from time to time.
6. Enjoy hot.

Low-FODMAP Glazed Brussels Sprouts

Prep: 15 minutes
Cook: 15 minutes
Total Time: 30 minutes
Serving portions: 4

Nutrition facts:
Calories 86, Total Fat 3.7 g, Saturated Fat 3 g, Cholesterol 0 mg, Sodium 507 mg,
Total Carbs 12.1 g, Fiber 2.8 g, Sugar 5.1 g, Protein 3.1 g

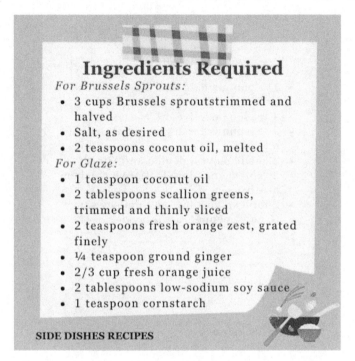

Ingredients Required

For Brussels Sprouts:
- 3 cups Brussels sproutstrimmed and halved
- Salt, as desired
- 2 teaspoons coconut oil, melted

For Glaze:
- 1 teaspoon coconut oil
- 2 tablespoons scallion greens, trimmed and thinly sliced
- 2 teaspoons fresh orange zest, grated finely
- ¼ teaspoon ground ginger
- 2/3 cup fresh orange juice
- 2 tablespoons low-sodium soy sauce
- 1 teaspoon cornstarch

SIDE DISHES RECIPES

Procedure of Cooking

1. Preheat your oven to 400 °F.
2. Arrange a baking paper into a roasting pan.
3. In a bowl, put in Brussels sprouts, a little salt, and oil. Toss to blend.
4. Put the Brussels sprouts mixture into the roasting pan.
5. Roast for about 10-15 minutes, flipping once halfway through.
6. Meanwhile, for glaze: in a flat-bottomed wok, add the coconut oil and let in melt on the burner on medium heat.
7. Cook the scallion greens for almost 2-3 minutes.
8. Add in the orange zest and cook for about 1 minute.
9. Put in ginger, orange juice, and soy sauce. Cook for almost 5 minutes.
10. Slowly put in the tapioca starch, beating regularly.
11. Cook for about 2-3 minutes more, stirring regularly.
12. Add the salt and remove from burner.
13. Put the roasted Brussels sprouts to a serving plate and top with orange glaze evenly.
14. Enjoy immediately.

Low-FODMAP Spinach with Mushrooms

Prep: 15 minutes
Cook: 15 minutes
Total Time: 30 minutes
Serving portions: 4

Nutrition facts:
Calories 63, Total Fat 4 g, Saturated Fat 0.5 g, Cholesterol 0 mg, Sodium 81 mg, Total Carbs 5.5 g, Fiber 2.3 g, Sugar 1.9 g, Protein 4.2 g

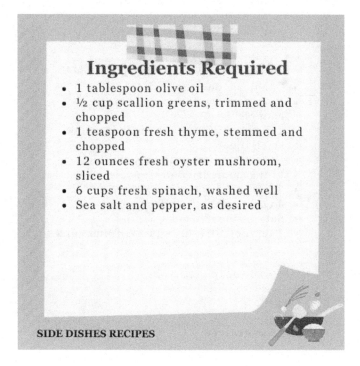

Ingredients Required

- 1 tablespoon olive oil
- ½ cup scallion greens, trimmed and chopped
- 1 teaspoon fresh thyme, stemmed and chopped
- 12 ounces fresh oyster mushroom, sliced
- 6 cups fresh spinach, washed well
- Sea salt and pepper, as desired

SIDE DISHES RECIPES

Procedure of Cooking

1. In a large-sized, flat-bottomed wok, put oil on the burner and sizzle at medium heat.
2. Cook the scallion greens for about 3-4 minutes.
3. Put in the thyme and cook for 1 minute.
4. Add the mushrooms and cook for about 5-6 minutes.
5. Put in the spinach and cook for about 3-4 minutes.
6. Add in the salt and pepper. Enjoy hot.

Low-FODMAP Zucchini with Tomatoes

Prep: 15 minutes
Cook: 17 minutes
Total Time: 32 minutes
Serving portions: 6

Nutrition facts:
Calories 72, Total Fat 5 g, Saturated Fat 0.7 g, Cholesterol 0 mg, Sodium 39 mg, Total Carbs 7 g, Fiber 2.2 g, Sugar 4.1 g, Protein 1.8 g

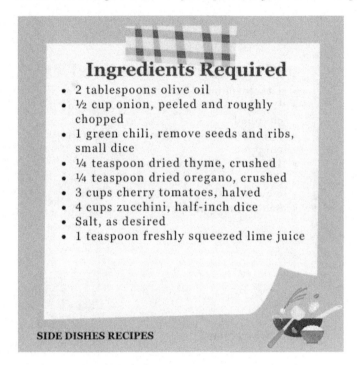

Ingredients Required
- 2 tablespoons olive oil
- ½ cup onion, peeled and roughly chopped
- 1 green chili, remove seeds and ribs, small dice
- ¼ teaspoon dried thyme, crushed
- ¼ teaspoon dried oregano, crushed
- 3 cups cherry tomatoes, halved
- 4 cups zucchini, half-inch dice
- Salt, as desired
- 1 teaspoon freshly squeezed lime juice

SIDE DISHES RECIPES

Procedure of Cooking

1. In a flat-bottomed wok, put oil on burner and sizzle at medium heat.
2. Cook onion for about 3-4 minutes.
3. Add green chili and dried herbs. Cook for almost 1 minute.
4. Add zucchini and cook for about 3-4 minutes.
5. Add tomatoes and salt. Cook for about 7-8 minutes.
6. Put in lime juice and enjoy hot.

Low-FODMAP Zucchini Noodles with Tomatoes

Prep: 15 minutes
Cook: 6 minutes
Total Time: 21 minutes
Serving portions: 3

Nutrition facts:
Calories 112, Total Fat 9.7 g, Saturated Fat 1.4 g, Cholesterol 0 mg, Sodium 66 mg,
Total Carbs 6.7 g, Fiber 2.2 g, Sugar 3.8 g, Protein 2.1 g

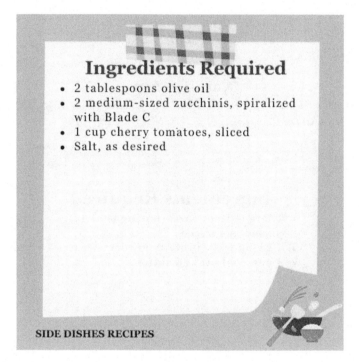

Ingredients Required

- 2 tablespoons olive oil
- 2 medium-sized zucchinis, spiralized with Blade C
- 1 cup cherry tomatoes, sliced
- Salt, as desired

SIDE DISHES RECIPES

Procedure of Cooking

1. In a flat-bottomed wok, put oil on burner at medium heat.
2. Cook zucchini for 3 minutes.
3. Put in the cherry tomatoes and salt. Cook for about 2-3 minutes.
4. Enjoy hot.

SMOOTHIES & DRINKS RECIPES

Low-FODMAP Coffee Smoothie

Prep: 10 minutes
Total time: 10 minutes
Serving portions: 2

Nutrition facts:
Calories 120, Total Fat 1.1 g, Saturated Fat 0.5 g, Cholesterol 31 mg, Sodium 30 mg, Total Carbs 17.3 g, Fiber 1.8 g, Sugar 8.8 g, Protein 11.6 g

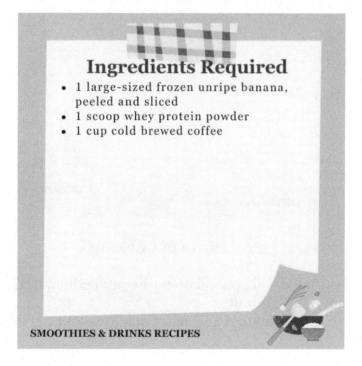

Ingredients Required
- 1 large-sized frozen unripe banana, peeled and sliced
- 1 scoop whey protein powder
- 1 cup cold brewed coffee

SMOOTHIES & DRINKS RECIPES

Procedure of Cooking

1. In a high-power processor, put banana, protein powder, and coffee. Process until creamy.
2. Pour the smoothie into your glasses and enjoy.

Low-FODMAP Banana Smoothie

Prep: 10 minutes
Total Time: 10 minutes
Serving portions: 2

Nutrition facts:
Calories 159, Total Fat 3.2 g, Saturated Fat 0.4 g, Cholesterol 0 mg, Sodium 1711 mg, Total Carbs 33.2 g, Fiber 4.5 g, Sugar 17 g, Protein 2.3 g

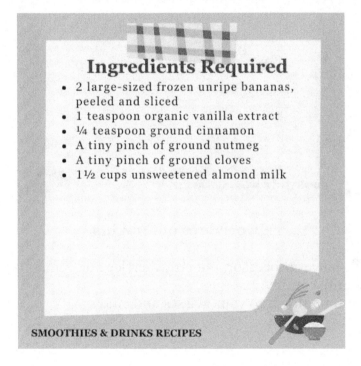

Ingredients Required

- 2 large-sized frozen unripe bananas, peeled and sliced
- 1 teaspoon organic vanilla extract
- ¼ teaspoon ground cinnamon
- A tiny pinch of ground nutmeg
- A tiny pinch of ground cloves
- 1½ cups unsweetened almond milk

SMOOTHIES & DRINKS RECIPES

Procedure of Cooking

1. In a high-power processor, put banana and remaining ingredients. Process until creamy.
2. Pour the smoothie into your glasses and enjoy.

Low-FODMAP Strawberry Smoothie

Prep: 10 minutes
Total Time: 10 minutes
Serving portions: 2

Nutrition facts:
Calories 129, Total Fat 4 g, Saturated Fat 0.4 g, Cholesterol 0 mg, Sodium 182 mg,
Total Carbs 23.9 g, Fiber 4.7 g, Sugar 12.6 g, Protein 2.4 g

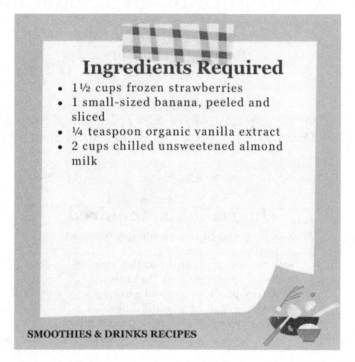

Ingredients Required

- 1½ cups frozen strawberries
- 1 small-sized banana, peeled and sliced
- ¼ teaspoon organic vanilla extract
- 2 cups chilled unsweetened almond milk

SMOOTHIES & DRINKS RECIPES

Procedure of Cooking

1. In a high-power processor, put strawberries and remaining ingredients. Process until creamy.
2. Pour the smoothie into your glasses and enjoy.

Low-FODMAP Pineapple Smoothie

Prep: 10 minutes
Total time: 10 minutes
Serving portions: 2

Nutrition facts:
Calories 90, Total Fat 0.7 g, Saturated Fat 0.1 g, Cholesterol 0 mg, Sodium 2 mg,
Total Carbs 22.8 g, Fiber 2.9 g, Sugar 16.3 g, Protein 1.2 g

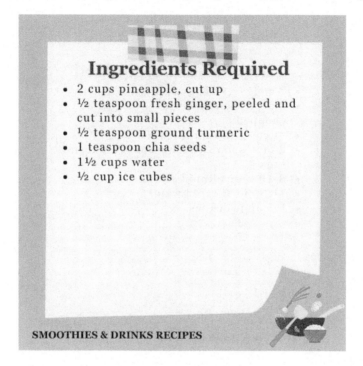

Ingredients Required

- 2 cups pineapple, cut up
- ½ teaspoon fresh ginger, peeled and cut into small pieces
- ½ teaspoon ground turmeric
- 1 teaspoon chia seeds
- 1½ cups water
- ½ cup ice cubes

SMOOTHIES & DRINKS RECIPES

Procedure of Cooking

1. Into a high-power processor, put pineapple and remaining ingredients. Process until creamy.
2. Pour the smoothie into your glasses and enjoy.

Low-FODMAP Spinach Smoothie

Prep: 10 minutes
Total Time: 10 minutes
Serving portions: 2

Nutrition facts:
Calories 23, Total Fat 0.4 g, Saturated Fat 0.2 g, Cholesterol 0 mg, Sodium 33 mg,
Total Carbs 4 g, Fiber 1.9 g, Sugar 1 g, Protein 1.6 g

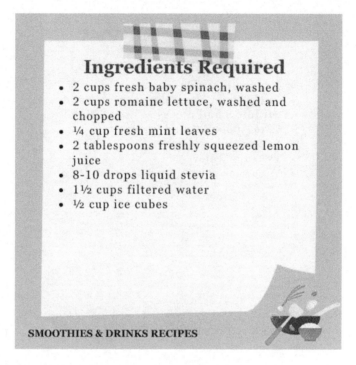

Ingredients Required

- 2 cups fresh baby spinach, washed
- 2 cups romaine lettuce, washed and chopped
- ¼ cup fresh mint leaves
- 2 tablespoons freshly squeezed lemon juice
- 8-10 drops liquid stevia
- 1½ cups filtered water
- ½ cup ice cubes

SMOOTHIES & DRINKS RECIPES

Procedure of Cooking

1. Into a high-power food processor, put spinach and remaining ingredients. Process until creamy.
2. Pour the smoothie into your glasses and enjoy.

Low-FODMAP Orange Juice

Prep: 10 minutes
Total Time: 10 minutes
Serving portions: 4

Nutrition facts:
Calories 113, Total Fat 0.2 g, Saturated Fat 0 g, Cholesterol 0 mg, Sodium 1 mg,
Total Carbs 28.3 g, Fiber 4.4 g, Sugar 23.2 g, Protein 1.7 g

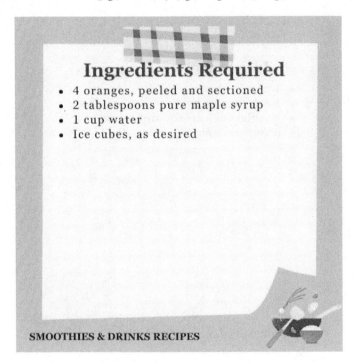

Ingredients Required

- 4 oranges, peeled and sectioned
- 2 tablespoons pure maple syrup
- 1 cup water
- Ice cubes, as desired

SMOOTHIES & DRINKS RECIPES

Procedure of Cooking

1. Place the orange sections, maple syrup, and water into a high-power blender and process until perfectly smooth.
2. Divide the ice cubes into your glasses.
3. Through a fine mesh strainer, strain the juice and pour it into glasses over ice.
4. Enjoy immediately.

Low-FODMAP Strawberry Detox Water

Prep: 10 minutes
Total Time: 10 minutes
Serving portions: 3

Nutrition facts:
Calories 18, Total Fat 0.2 g, Saturated Fat 0 g, Cholesterol 0 mg, Sodium 1 mg,
Total Carbs 4.3 g, Fiber 1.2 g, Sugar 2.5 g, Protein 0.4 g

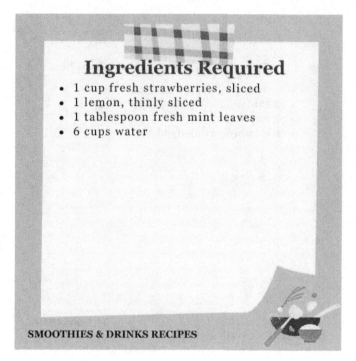

Ingredients Required
- 1 cup fresh strawberries, sliced
- 1 lemon, thinly sliced
- 1 tablespoon fresh mint leaves
- 6 cups water

SMOOTHIES & DRINKS RECIPES

Procedure of Cooking

1. In a large-sized glass jar, place strawberry, lemon, and mint leaves. Pour water on top.
2. Cover the jar with a lid and put in your refrigerator for 2-4 hours before enjoying it.

Low-FODMAP Lemonade

Prep: 10 minutes
Total Time: 10 minutes
Serving portions: 4

Nutrition facts:
Calories 11, Total Fat 0.4 g, Saturated Fat 0.4 g, Cholesterol 0 mg, Sodium 9 mg, Total Carbs 1 g, Fiber 0.2 g, Sugar 1 g, Protein 0.4 g

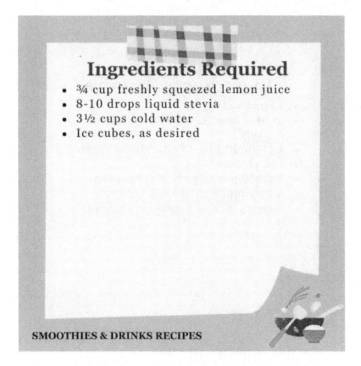

Ingredients Required
- ¾ cup freshly squeezed lemon juice
- 8-10 drops liquid stevia
- 3½ cups cold water
- Ice cubes, as desired

SMOOTHIES & DRINKS RECIPES

Procedure of Cooking

1. In a large-sized pitcher, blend together the lemon juice and stevia.
2. Add in the water and add ice to fill the pitcher.
3. Enjoy chilled.

Low-FODMAP Lemony Ginger Tea

Prep: 10 minutes
Cook: 15 minutes
Total Time: 25 minutes
Serving portions: 4

Nutrition facts:
Calories 29, Total Fat 0.1 g, Saturated Fat 0 g, Cholesterol 0 mg, Sodium 1 mg,
Total Carbs 7.3 g, Fiber 0.2 g, Sugar 6 g, Protein 0.1 g

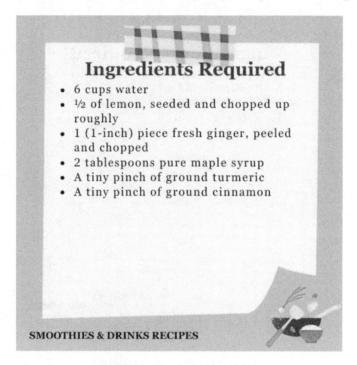

Ingredients Required

- 6 cups water
- ½ of lemon, seeded and chopped up roughly
- 1 (1-inch) piece fresh ginger, peeled and chopped
- 2 tablespoons pure maple syrup
- A tiny pinch of ground turmeric
- A tiny pinch of ground cinnamon

SMOOTHIES & DRINKS RECIPES

Procedure of Cooking

1. In a saucepan, put in water and remaining ingredients on the burner at medium-high heat and cook until boiling.
2. Adjust the heat to medium-low and cook for about 10-12 minutes.
3. Strain into cups and enjoy hot.

Low-FODMAP Hot Apple Cider

Prep: 10 minutes
Cook: 25 minutes
Total Time: 35 minutes
Serving portions: 4

Nutrition facts:
Calories 119, Total Fat 0.1 g, Saturated Fat 0.1 g, Cholesterol 0 mg, Sodium 6 mg, Total Carbs 28.4 g, Fiber 0.7 g, Sugar 26.1 g, Protein 0.1 g

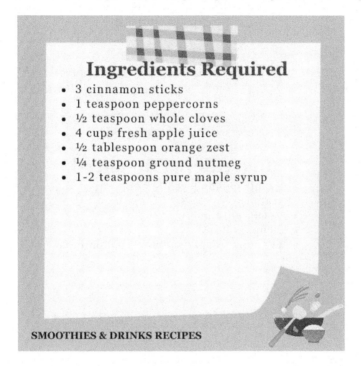

Ingredients Required

- 3 cinnamon sticks
- 1 teaspoon peppercorns
- ½ teaspoon whole cloves
- 4 cups fresh apple juice
- ½ tablespoon orange zest
- ¼ teaspoon ground nutmeg
- 1-2 teaspoons pure maple syrup

SMOOTHIES & DRINKS RECIPES

Procedure of Cooking

1. Put an anti-sticking saucepan on the burner and sizzle at medium-high heat.
2. Toast the cinnamon sticks, peppercorns, and cloves for about 3-5 minutes, stirring regularly.
3. Put in the apple juice, orange zest, and nutmeg. Cook until boiling.
4. Adjust the heat to low and cook for about 15-20 minutes.
5. Through a fine-mesh sieve, strain the mixture into serving mugs and enjoy.

DESSERT RECIPES

Low-FODMAP Lemon Sorbet

Prep: 10 minutes
Total Time: 10 minutes
Serving portions: 4

Nutrition facts:
Calories 185, Total Fat 2.8 g, Saturated Fat 2.7 g , Cholesterol 0 mg, Sodium 74 mg, Total Carbs 34.1 g, Fiber 1.5 g, Sugar 30.7 g, Protein 2.8 g

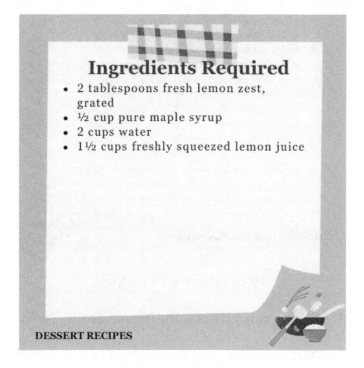

Ingredients Required
- 2 tablespoons fresh lemon zest, grated
- ½ cup pure maple syrup
- 2 cups water
- 1½ cups freshly squeezed lemon juice

DESSERT RECIPES

Procedure of Cooking

1. Freeze ice cream maker tub for almost 24 hours before making this sorbet.
2. Put lemon zest, maple syrup, and water in a saucepan on burner and cook at medium heat for about 1 minute, stirring regularly.
3. Take off the pan from burner and blend in the lemon juice.
4. Immediately place this sorbet into the ice cream maker tub and put in your refrigerator for 2 hours.

Low-FODMAP Raspberry Mousse

Prep: 10 minutes
Total time: 10 minutes
Serving portions: 4

Nutrition facts:
Calories 44, Total Fat 0.8 g, Saturated Fat 0.1 g, Cholesterol 0 mg, Sodium 164 mg, Total Carbs 9.4 g, Fiber 5.1 g, Sugar 3.5 g, Protein 1 g

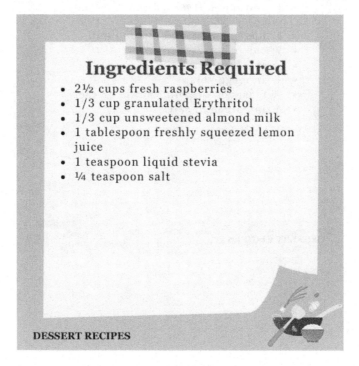

Ingredients Required
- 2½ cups fresh raspberries
- 1/3 cup granulated Erythritol
- 1/3 cup unsweetened almond milk
- 1 tablespoon freshly squeezed lemon juice
- 1 teaspoon liquid stevia
- ¼ teaspoon salt

DESSERT RECIPES

Procedure of Cooking

1. In a clean food processor, put raspberries and remaining ingredients. Process until perfectly smooth.
2. Put the blended mixture into serving glasses and put in your refrigerator to chill before enjoying.

Low-FODMAP Blueberry Gelato

Prep: 15 minutes
Cook: 10 minutes
Total Time: 25 minutes
Serving portions: 6

Nutrition facts:
Calories 89, Total Fat 6.2 g, Saturated Fat 2.4 g, Cholesterol 147 mg, Sodium 95 mg, Total Carbs 6.6 g, Fiber 1.2 g, Sugar 3.8 g, Protein 2.5 g

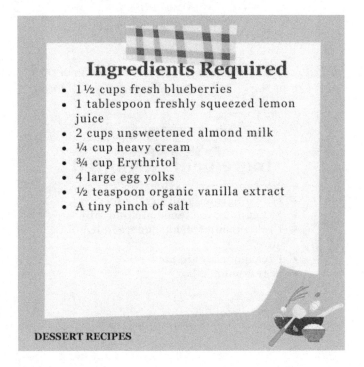

Ingredients Required

- 1½ cups fresh blueberries
- 1 tablespoon freshly squeezed lemon juice
- 2 cups unsweetened almond milk
- ¼ cup heavy cream
- ¾ cup Erythritol
- 4 large egg yolks
- ½ teaspoon organic vanilla extract
- A tiny pinch of salt

DESSERT RECIPES

Procedure of Cooking

1. In a clean food processor, put blueberries and lemon juice. Process until perfectly smooth.
2. Through a fine sieve, strain the blueberry mixture into a bowl by pressing with the back of a wooden spoon.
3. Discard the peel and set the puree aside.
4. In a saucepan, put milk and cream on the burner at medium heat and cook until boiling.
5. Take off the saucepan of milk mixture from burner and set it aside.
6. In a bowl, put in sugar and egg yolks and, with an electric mixer, beat until yellow, pale, and thick.
7. Add ¼ of the hot milk mixture and whisk until smooth.
8. Put the mixture into the pan with remaining milk mixture.
9. Return the pan on the burner at low heat and cook for 4 minutes, stirring regularly.
10. Take off the pan of milk mixture from burner and immediately strain into a bowl.
11. Immediately add in vanilla extract, salt, and strained blueberry puree.
12. Put in your refrigerator, covered, overnight.
13. Put the blueberry mixture into an ice cream maker and freeze according to manufacturer's directions.
14. Put the ice cream into a sealable container and freeze until set completely.

Low-FODMAP Cottage Cheese Pudding

Prep: 10 minutes
Cook: 35 minutes
Total Time: 45 minutes
Serving portions: 6

Nutrition facts:
Calories 119, Total Fat 8.5 g, Saturated Fat 4.6 g, Cholesterol 105 mg, Sodium 190 mg, Total Carbs 2.1 g, Fiber 0 g, Sugar 0.4 g, Protein 8.3 g

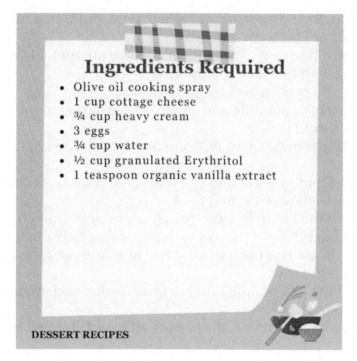

Ingredients Required

- Olive oil cooking spray
- 1 cup cottage cheese
- ¾ cup heavy cream
- 3 eggs
- ¾ cup water
- ½ cup granulated Erythritol
- 1 teaspoon organic vanilla extract

DESSERT RECIPES

Procedure of Cooking

1. Preheat your oven to 350 °F.
2. Grease six (6-ounce) ramekins with cooking spray.
3. In a clean food processor, put cottage cheese and remaining ingredients. Process until perfectly smooth.
4. Pour the blended mixture into the ramekins evenly.
5. Next, place ramekins into a large-sized baking dish.
6. Add hot water in the baking dish, about 1-inch up sides of the ramekins.
7. Cook it in your oven for 35 minutes.
8. Enjoy warm.

Low-FODMAP Spiced Egg Custard

Prep: 10 minutes
Cook: 40 minutes
Total Time: 50 minutes
Serving portions: 8

Nutrition facts:
Calories 103, Total Fat 3.8 g, Saturated Fat 1 g, Cholesterol 102 mg, Sodium 111 mg, Total Carbs 14.2 g, Fiber 0.4 g, Sugar 12 g, Protein 3.8 g

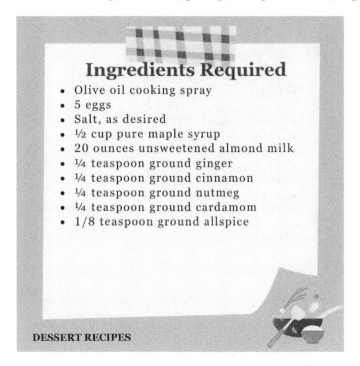

Ingredients Required

- Olive oil cooking spray
- 5 eggs
- Salt, as desired
- ½ cup pure maple syrup
- 20 ounces unsweetened almond milk
- ¼ teaspoon ground ginger
- ¼ teaspoon ground cinnamon
- ¼ teaspoon ground nutmeg
- ¼ teaspoon ground cardamom
- 1/8 teaspoon ground allspice

DESSERT RECIPES

Procedure of Cooking

1. Preheat your oven to 325 °F.
2. Grease eight (8) small ramekins with cooking spray.
3. In a bowl, put in the eggs and salt. Whisk well.
4. Arrange a fine-mesh sieve over a medium-sized bowl.
5. Through a sieve, strain the egg mixture into a bowl.
6. Pour maple syrup into the eggs and stir to blend.
7. Add in the almond milk and spices. Whisk until blended thoroughly.
8. Pour the blended mixture into the ramekins.
9. Next, place ramekins into a large-sized baking dish.
10. Add hot water in the baking dish about 2-inch high around the ramekins.
11. Cook it in your oven for about 30-40 minutes.
12. Take out ramekins from oven and set it aside to cool.
13. Put in your refrigerator to chill before enjoying.

Low-FODMAP Double Chocolate Cookies

Prep: 15 minutes
Cook: 11 minutes
Total Time: 26 minutes
Serving portions: 18

Nutrition facts:
Calories 141, Total Fat 11.1 g, Saturated Fat 2.4 g, Cholesterol 22 mg, Sodium 142 mg,
Total Carbs 8.7 g, Fiber 2.5 g, Sugar 5.5 g, Protein 4.8 g

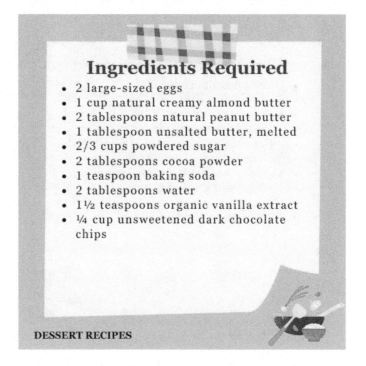

Ingredients Required
- 2 large-sized eggs
- 1 cup natural creamy almond butter
- 2 tablespoons natural peanut butter
- 1 tablespoon unsalted butter, melted
- 2/3 cups powdered sugar
- 2 tablespoons cocoa powder
- 1 teaspoon baking soda
- 2 tablespoons water
- 1½ teaspoons organic vanilla extract
- ¼ cup unsweetened dark chocolate chips

DESSERT RECIPES

Procedure of Cooking

1. Preheat your oven to 350°F.
2. Line a large-sized cookie sheet with baking paper.
3. In a large-sized bowl, padd in eggs and remaining ingredients, except chocolate chips, and, with an electric hand blender, mix until blended thoroughly.
4. Fold in the chocolate chips.
5. Make about 1½-inch balls from the dough and place onto the cookie sheet in a single layer, about 2-inch apart.
6. With your palm, flatten each ball slightly.
7. Bake in your oven for about 8-11 minutes.
8. Take the cookie sheet from oven and place onto a metal rack to cool for almost 5 minutes.
9. Carefully move the cookies onto the metal racks to cool thoroughly before enjoying them.

Low-FODMAP Coconut Macaroons

Prep: 15 minutes
Cook: 10 minutes
Total Time: 25 minutes
Serving portions: 12

Nutrition facts:
Calories 78, Total Fat 5.7 g, Saturated Fat 4.9 g, Cholesterol 0 mg, Sodium 26 mg, Total Carbs 6.5 g, Fiber 1 g, Sugar 4.7 g, Protein 0.4 g

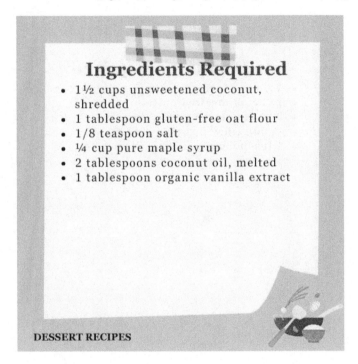

Ingredients Required

- 1½ cups unsweetened coconut, shredded
- 1 tablespoon gluten-free oat flour
- 1/8 teaspoon salt
- ¼ cup pure maple syrup
- 2 tablespoons coconut oil, melted
- 1 tablespoon organic vanilla extract

DESSERT RECIPES

Procedure of Cooking

1. Preheat your oven to 350°F.
2. Arrange baking paper to cover two large-sized cookie sheets.
3. In a clean food processor, put coconut and remaining ingredients. Process until blended thoroughly.
4. Divide the mixture into tablespoon-size portions and place them onto the cookie sheet.
5. Bake in your oven for about 7-10 minutes.
6. Remove the cookie sheet from oven and let the macaroons cool for almost 1 hour before enjoying them.

Low-FODMAP Peanut Butter Fudge

Prep: 10 minutes
Cook: 5 minutes
Total Time: 15 minutes
Serving portions: 16

Nutrition facts:
Calories 184, Total Fat 16 g, Saturated Fat 4.4 g, Cholesterol 14 mg, Sodium 91 mg,
Total Carbs 5.5 g, Fiber 1.5 g, Sugar 1.6 g, Protein 7.4 g

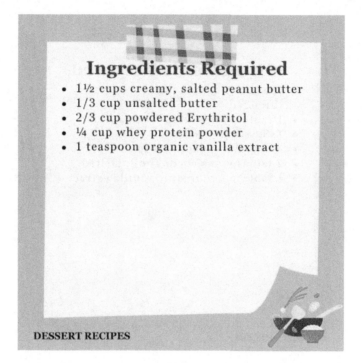

Ingredients Required

- 1½ cups creamy, salted peanut butter
- 1/3 cup unsalted butter
- 2/3 cup powdered Erythritol
- ¼ cup whey protein powder
- 1 teaspoon organic vanilla extract

DESSERT RECIPES

Procedure of Cooking

1. In a small-sized saucepan, put in peanut butter and butter on the burner at low heat and cook until melted and smooth.
2. Add in the Erythritol and protein powder. Blend until smooth.
3. Remove from burner and stir in vanilla extract.
4. Place the fudge mixture onto a paper-lined 8x8-inch baking dish and, with a spatula, smooth the top surface.
5. Freeze for about 30-45 minutes.
6. Carefully put the fudge onto a cutting board with the help of parchment paper.
7. Cut the fudge into equal-sized squares and enjoy.

Low-FODMAP Chocolate Banana Brownies

Prep: 15 minutes
Cook: 20 minutes
Total Time: 35 minutes
Serving portions: 12

Nutrition facts:
Calories 207, Total Fat 11.7 g, Saturated Fat 2.8 g, Cholesterol 0 mg, Sodium 164 mg, Total Carbs 19.9 g, Fiber 3.8 g, Sugar 9.5 g, Protein 10.7 g

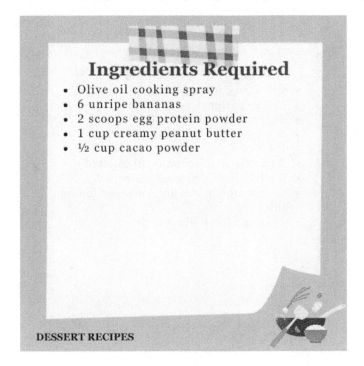

Ingredients Required

- Olive oil cooking spray
- 6 unripe bananas
- 2 scoops egg protein powder
- 1 cup creamy peanut butter
- ½ cup cacao powder

DESSERT RECIPES

Procedure of Cooking

1. Preheat your oven to 350°F.
2. Line a square baking dish with parchment paper and then grease it with cooking spray.
3. In a clean food processor, put bananas, protein powder, peanut butter, and cacao powder. Process until perfectly smooth.
4. Put the blended mixture into the baking dish evenly and, with the back of a spatula, smooth the top surface.
5. Bake it in your oven for about 18-20 minutes.
6. Take out the baking dish of brownies from oven and place onto a metal rack to cool thoroughly.
7. Cut into equal-sized brownies and enjoy.

Low-FODMAP Blueberry Crumble

Prep: 15 minutes
Cook: 40 minutes
Total Time: 55 minutes
Serving portions: 5

Nutrition facts:
Calories 129, Total Fat 6.4 g, Saturated Fat 4.7 g, Cholesterol 0 mg, Sodium 189 mg,
Total Carbs 16.8 g, Fiber 2.5 g, Sugar 5.3 g, Protein 2 g

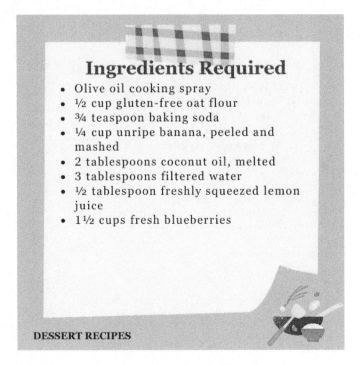

Ingredients Required

- Olive oil cooking spray
- ½ cup gluten-free oat flour
- ¾ teaspoon baking soda
- ¼ cup unripe banana, peeled and mashed
- 2 tablespoons coconut oil, melted
- 3 tablespoons filtered water
- ½ tablespoon freshly squeezed lemon juice
- 1½ cups fresh blueberries

DESSERT RECIPES

Procedure of Cooking

1. Preheat your oven to 300°F.
2. Lightly grease an 8x8-inch baking dish with cooking spray.
3. In a large-sized bowl, put in oat flour and remaining ingredients, except the blueberries, and stir until blended thoroughly.
4. In the bottom of the prepared baking dish, place the blueberries and top them with the flour mixture evenly.
5. Cook in your oven for 40 minutes.
6. Cut into squares and enjoy warm.

Low-FODMAP Curry Powder

Prep: 5 minutes
Total Time: 5 minutes
Serving portions: 20

Nutrition facts:
Calories 4, Total Fat 0.2 g, Saturated Fat 0 g, Cholesterol 0 mg, Sodium 1 mg,
Total Carbs 0.5 g, Fiber 0 g, Sugar 0.1 g, Protein 0.2 g

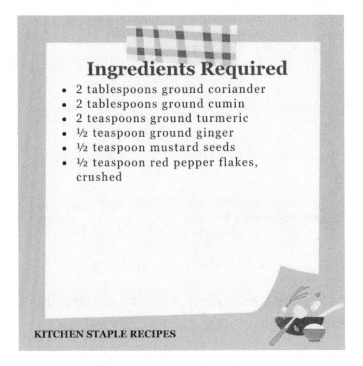

Ingredients Required
- 2 tablespoons ground coriander
- 2 tablespoons ground cumin
- 2 teaspoons ground turmeric
- ½ teaspoon ground ginger
- ½ teaspoon mustard seeds
- ½ teaspoon red pepper flakes, crushed

KITCHEN STAPLE RECIPES

Procedure of Cooking

1. Into a spice grinder, put in all spices and process until powdered finely.
2. Store in an airtight jar.

Low-FODMAP Italian Seasoning

Prep: 5 minutes
Total Time: 5 minutes
Serving portions: 16

Nutrition facts:
Calories 3, Total Fat 0.1 g, Saturated Fat 0 g, Cholesterol 0 mg, Sodium 148 mg,
Total Carbs 0.6 g, Fiber 0.3 g, Sugar 0.1 g, Protein 0.1 g

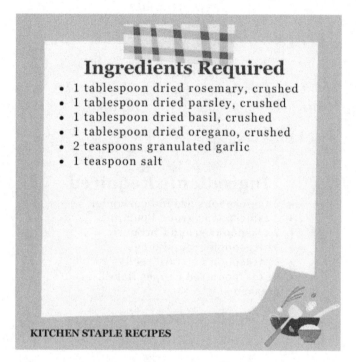

Ingredients Required
- 1 tablespoon dried rosemary, crushed
- 1 tablespoon dried parsley, crushed
- 1 tablespoon dried basil, crushed
- 1 tablespoon dried oregano, crushed
- 2 teaspoons granulated garlic
- 1 teaspoon salt

KITCHEN STAPLE RECIPES

Procedure of Cooking

1. In a bowl, blend together dried herbs, garlic, and salt.
2. Store in airtight jar.

Low-FODMAP Taco Seasoning

Prep: 5 minutes
Total Time: 5 minutes
Serving portions: 10

Nutrition facts:
Calories 8, Total Fat 0.4 g, Saturated Fat 0 g, Cholesterol 0 mg, Sodium 25 mg, Total Carbs 1.1 g, Fiber 0.5 g, Sugar 0.1 g, Protein 0.4 g

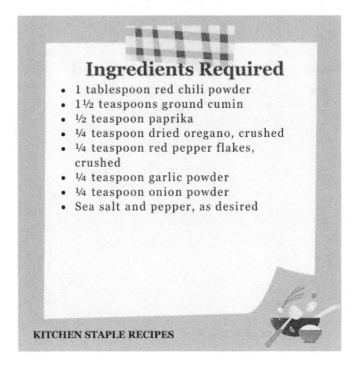

Ingredients Required
- 1 tablespoon red chili powder
- 1½ teaspoons ground cumin
- ½ teaspoon paprika
- ¼ teaspoon dried oregano, crushed
- ¼ teaspoon red pepper flakes, crushed
- ¼ teaspoon garlic powder
- ¼ teaspoon onion powder
- Sea salt and pepper, as desired

KITCHEN STAPLE RECIPES

Procedure of Cooking

1. In a small-sized bowl, put in chili powder and remaining ingredients. Stir thoroughly.

2. Store in an airtight jar.

Low-FODMAP Ginger-Garlic Paste

Prep: 10 minutes
Total Time: 10 minutes
Serving portions: 24

Nutrition facts:
Calories 15, Total Fat 0.7 g, Saturated Fat 0.1 g, Cholesterol 0 mg, Sodium 1 mg,
Total Carbs 2.1 g, Fiber 0.2 g, Sugar 0.1 g, Protein 0.4 g

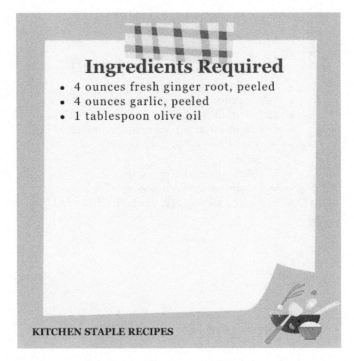

Ingredients Required
- 4 ounces fresh ginger root, peeled
- 4 ounces garlic, peeled
- 1 tablespoon olive oil

KITCHEN STAPLE RECIPES

Procedure of Cooking

1. Into a clean food processor, put ginger and garlic. Process until finely chopped.
2. Slowly add oil and process until perfectly smooth.
3. Put the paste into an airtight jar and store in your refrigerator.

Low-FODMAP Prepared Mustard

Prep: 10 minutes
Total Time: 10 minutes
Serving portions: 12

Nutrition facts:
Calories 41, Total Fat 2 g, Saturated Fat 0.2 g, Cholesterol 0 mg, Sodium 14 mg,
Total Carbs 4.5 g, Fiber 1 g, Sugar 2.4 g, Protein 1.7 g

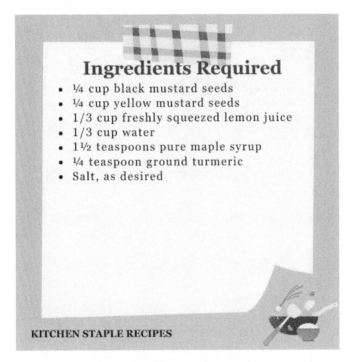

Ingredients Required
- ¼ cup black mustard seeds
- ¼ cup yellow mustard seeds
- 1/3 cup freshly squeezed lemon juice
- 1/3 cup water
- 1½ teaspoons pure maple syrup
- ¼ teaspoon ground turmeric
- Salt, as desired

KITCHEN STAPLE RECIPES

Procedure of Cooking

1. In a large-sized, glass bowl, blend together mustard seeds, lemon juice. and water. Set it aside, covered, for about 24-36 hours.
2. Into a high-power processor, add mustard seeds mixture and remaining ingredients. Process until perfectly smooth.
3. Put the mustard into an airtight jar and store in your refrigerator.

Low-FODMAP Peanut Butter

Prep: 10 minutes
Total Time: 10 minutes
Serving portions: 16

Nutrition facts:
Calories 107, Total Fat 9 g, Saturated Fat 1.3 g, Cholesterol 0 mg, Sodium 15 mg, Total Carbs 3.8 g, Fiber 1.6 g, Sugar 1.5 g, Protein 4.7 g

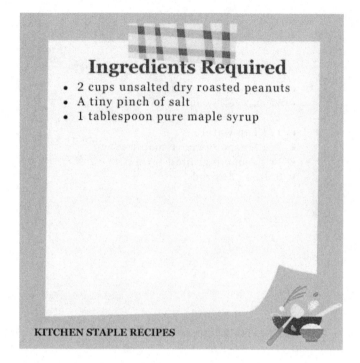

Ingredients Required

- 2 cups unsalted dry roasted peanuts
- A tiny pinch of salt
- 1 tablespoon pure maple syrup

KITCHEN STAPLE RECIPES

Procedure of Cooking

1. In a clean food processor, put peanuts and salt. Process for 5 minutes.
2. Add maple syrup and process until just blended.
3. Put the peanut butter into an airtight container and store in your refrigerator.

Low-FODMAP Mayonnaise

Prep: 10 minutes
Total Time: 10 minutes
Serving portions: 10

Nutrition facts:
Calories 193, Total Fat 22 g, Saturated Fat 11.2 g, Cholesterol 42 mg, Sodium 2 mg, Total Carbs 0.3 g, Fiber 0.1 g, Sugar 0.1 g, Protein 0.6 g

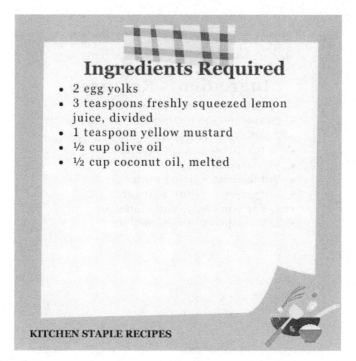

Ingredients Required

- 2 egg yolks
- 3 teaspoons freshly squeezed lemon juice, divided
- 1 teaspoon yellow mustard
- ½ cup olive oil
- ½ cup coconut oil, melted

KITCHEN STAPLE RECIPES

Procedure of Cooking

1. In a clean processor, put egg yolks, 1 tablespoon of lemon juice, and mustard. Process until blended.
2. Next, slowly add in both oils and process until a thick mixture forms.
3. Put in remaining lemon juice, salt, and pepper. Process until blended thoroughly.

Low-FODMAP Worcestershire Sauce

Prep: 5 minutes
Cook: 4 minutes
Total Time: 9 minutes
Serving portions: 10

Nutrition facts:
Calories 5, Total Fat 0 g, Saturated Fat 0 g, Cholesterol 0 mg, Sodium 177 mg,
Total Carbs 0.5 g, Fiber 0.1 g, Sugar 0.3 g, Protein 0.2 g

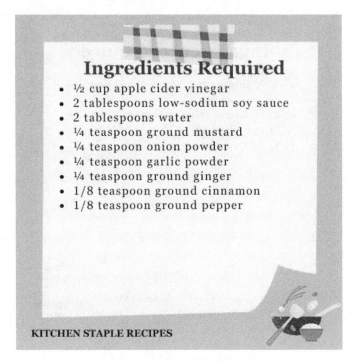

Ingredients Required

- ½ cup apple cider vinegar
- 2 tablespoons low-sodium soy sauce
- 2 tablespoons water
- ¼ teaspoon ground mustard
- ¼ teaspoon onion powder
- ¼ teaspoon garlic powder
- ¼ teaspoon ground ginger
- 1/8 teaspoon ground cinnamon
- 1/8 teaspoon ground pepper

KITCHEN STAPLE RECIPES

Procedure of Cooking

1. In a small-sized saucepan, blend together vinegar and remaining ingredients on the burner at medium heat and cook until boiling.
2. Next, adjust the heat to low and cook for about 1-2 minutes.
3. Take the pan of sauce from burner and set it aside to cool thoroughly.
4. Put the sauce into an airtight glass jar and store in your refrigerator for about 4-6 months.

Low-FODMAP BBQ Sauce

Prep: 10 minutes
Cook: 20 minutes
Total Time: 30 minutes
Serving portions: 16

Nutrition facts:
Calories 24, Total Fat 0.4 g, Saturated Fat 0 g, Cholesterol 502 mg, Sodium 0 mg,
Total Carbs 5.3 g, Fiber 1 g, Sugar 3.7 g, Protein 0.4 g

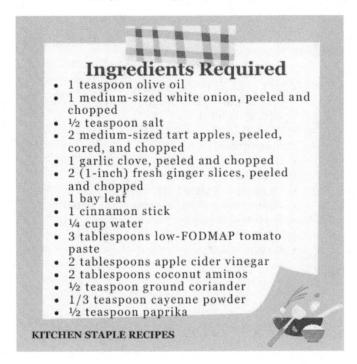

Ingredients Required
- 1 teaspoon olive oil
- 1 medium-sized white onion, peeled and chopped
- ½ teaspoon salt
- 2 medium-sized tart apples, peeled, cored, and chopped
- 1 garlic clove, peeled and chopped
- 2 (1-inch) fresh ginger slices, peeled and chopped
- 1 bay leaf
- 1 cinnamon stick
- ¼ cup water
- 3 tablespoons low-FODMAP tomato paste
- 2 tablespoons apple cider vinegar
- 2 tablespoons coconut aminos
- ½ teaspoon ground coriander
- 1/3 teaspoon cayenne powder
- ½ teaspoon paprika

KITCHEN STAPLE RECIPES

Procedure of Cooking

1. In a large-sized saucepan, put oil on the burner and sizzle at medium heat.
2. Cook onion and salt for about 2-3 minutes.
3. Add apples, garlic, ginger, and bay leaf. Cook for 2 minutes.
4. Put in remaining ingredients and cook until boiling.
5. Next, adjust the heat to low and cook, covered, for 15 minutes, stirring from time to time.
6. Take the pan of sauce from burner and let it cool slightly.
7. Discard the ginger, bay leaf, and cinnamon stick.
8. Put the sauce mixture into a clean food processor and process until perfectly smooth.
9. Next, strain the mixture through a fine sieve, pressing with the back of a spoon.
10. Put the sauce into an airtight jar and store in the refrigerator.

Low-FODMAP Chicken Broth

Prep: 15 minutes
Cook: 2 hours
Total Time: 2¼ hours
Serving portions: 8

Nutrition facts:
Calories 288, Total Fat 10.6 g, Saturated Fat 2.9 g, Cholesterol 126 mg,
Sodium 137 mg, Total Carbs 4.3 g, Fiber 1.1 g, Sugar 2 g, Protein 41.5 g

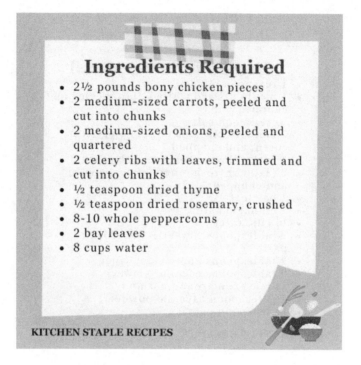

Ingredients Required

- 2½ pounds bony chicken pieces
- 2 medium-sized carrots, peeled and cut into chunks
- 2 medium-sized onions, peeled and quartered
- 2 celery ribs with leaves, trimmed and cut into chunks
- ½ teaspoon dried thyme
- ½ teaspoon dried rosemary, crushed
- 8-10 whole peppercorns
- 2 bay leaves
- 8 cups water

KITCHEN STAPLE RECIPES

Procedure of Cooking

1. In a large-sized Dutch oven, place chicken pieces and remaining ingredients on the burner at high heat and cook until boiling.
2. Next, adjust the heat to low and cook, covered, for 2 hours, skimming foam from the top from time to time.
3. Remove the pan of broth from burner and, through a fine mesh strainer, strain the broth.
4. Set the strained broth aside to cool thoroughly at room temperature.
5. Place the cooled broth into a container and put in your refrigerator overnight.
6. Carefully discard the solidified fat from the top of the chilled broth.
7. You can preserve this broth in your refrigerator for 3 days or up to 3-4 months in the freezer.

MEASUREMENT CONVERSION

Volume Equivalent (Dry)

METRIC	US STANDARDS (Approximate)
0.5 ml	1/8 teaspoon
1 ml	¼ teaspoon
2 ml	½ teaspoon
4 ml	1 teaspoon
15 ml	¼ cup
59 ml	½ cup
118 ml	¾ cup
177 ml	1 cup
235 ml	2 cups
700 ml	3 cups
1 L	4 cups

Volume Equivalent (Liquid)

US STANDARDS	METRIC (Approximate)	US STANDARDS (ounces)
2 tablespoons	30 ml	1 fl oz.
¼ cup	60 ml	2 fl. oz
½ cup	120 ml	4 fl oz.
1 cup	240 ml	8 fl. oz.
1 ½ cup	355 ml	12 fl oz.
1 pint or 2 cups	475	16 fl. oz.
1 quart or 4 cups	1 L	32 fl. oz.
1 gallon	4 L	128 fl. oz.

Weight Equivalents

METRIC	US STANDARDS
28g	1 ounce
57g	2 ounces
142g	5 ounces
284g	10 ounces
425g	15 ounces
455g	16 ounces (1 lb.)
680g	1 ½ pound
907g	2 pounds

CONCLUSION

As we reach the end of this low-FODMAP recipes cookbook, I hope that it has served as a valuable resource in your journey towards better digestive health and overall well-being. Throughout these pages, I have strived to present a diverse range of recipes that are both satisfying and safe for those with sensitive digestive systems. From breakfast to dinner, from snacks to desserts, I have explored a multitude of flavors and ingredients that will inspire your creativity in the kitchen.

I understand that embracing a low-FODMAP lifestyle can initially feel overwhelming, with its long lists of foods to avoid and the challenge of finding suitable alternatives. However, I hope that this cookbook has empowered you to take control of your diet and discover a new world of culinary possibilities. By focusing on low-FODMAP ingredients and mindful cooking techniques, you can still enjoy a rich and varied diet without sacrificing taste or nutrition. Remember, everyone's journey with food is unique, and it may take some time to find the perfect balance of ingredients that work for you. Don't be discouraged by setbacks or experimentation—every step is a valuable learning experience. Embrace the process of discovering which foods fuel your body and bring you joy, and be patient with yourself along the way. May this cookbook continue to be a source of inspiration and support as you embrace the world of low-FODMAP cooking. Wishing you good health, happiness, and many delicious meals to come.

Notes

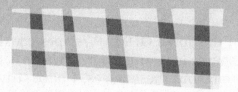

Notes

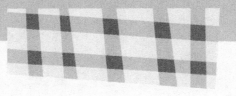

Notes

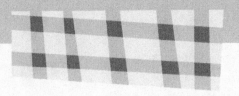

Notes

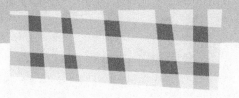

Notes

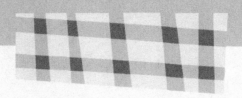

Notes

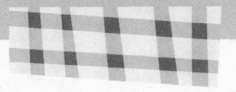

Notes

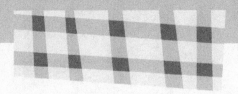

Notes

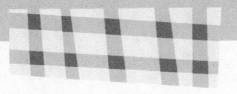

Notes

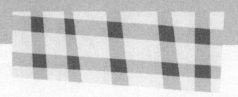

Made in United States
North Haven, CT
13 September 2023

41521441R00083